Neurologic Disorders in Pregnancy

Neurologic Disorders in Pregnancy

Edited by

Jacqueline M. Washington MD

Department of Neurology, Emory University School of Medicine
Atlanta, Georgia, USA

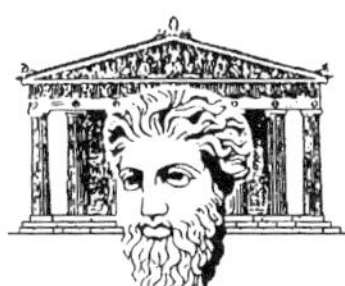

The Parthenon Publishing Group

International Publishers in Medicine, Science & Technology

A CRC PRESS COMPANY

BOCA RATON LONDON NEW YORK WASHINGTON, D.C.

Published in the USA by
The Parthenon Publishing Group
345 Park Avenue South, 10th Floor
New York, NY 10010
USA

Published in the UK and Europe by
The Parthenon Publishing Group
23–25 Blades Court
Deodar Road
London SW15 2NU
UK

Library of Congress Cataloging-in-Publication Data

Data available on request

British Library Cataloguing in Publication Data

Data available on request

ISBN 1-84214-189-9

Typeset by Martin Lister Publishing Services, Carnforth, Lancs, UK
Printed and bound by Antony Rowe Ltd., Chippenham, Wiltshire, UK

Contents

List of principal contributors

C. B. Britton
Columbia University
Neurological Insititute
710 W. 168th Street
New York, NY 10032-2603
USA

P. K. Coyle
SUNY at Stony Brook
Department of Neurology
Health Sciences Center T12
Stony Brook, NY 11794-8121
USA

J. M. Gilchrist
Brown Medical School
593 Eddy Street
APC 689
Providence, RI 02903
USA

J. M. Massey
Duke University Medical Center
Division of Neurology
PO Box 3403
Duke South Clinic 1L
Durham, NC 27710
USA

P. B. Pennell
Emory University School of Medicine
Emory Epilepsy Monitoring Unit
1639 Pierce Drive
Atlanta, GA 30322
USA

S. D. Silberstein
Thomas Jefferson University Hospital
Jefferson Headache Center
111 South 11th Street
Philadelphia, PA 19107
USA

B. J. Stern
Emory University School of Medicine
Department of Neurology
1365 Clifton Road
Atlanta, GA 30322
USA

S. Waddy
Emory University School of Medicine
Department of Neurology
1365 Clifton Road
Atlanta GA, 30322
USA

J. M. Washington
Emory University School of Medicine
Department of Neurology
1365 Clifton Road
Atlanta, GA 30322
USA

Preface

The past 20 years have witnessed remarkable developments and insights into the treatment of neurologic disorders in pregnancy. The patient, practitioners, therapies and prognosis of neurologic disease have all changed. Today's patient is on average older, better informed and more involved in her own health care. Practitioners are more likely to consider pregnancy and potential pregnancy when making decisions regarding therapy. These past 20 years have heralded the development of novel therapies for many neurologic diseases; many novel agents in the treatment of epilepsy, multiple sclerosis, myasthenia gravis and headache have been developed over this period of time. This book was written to promote improved understanding and up-to-date therapy, with recent developments and insights in mind.

Neurologic Disorders of Pregnancy is a work designed to bridge gaps in understanding. The first bridge allows us to travel from treatment 20 years ago to expanded understanding and current therapy. The second bridge is located in that black box of medicine. Neurology and obstetrics in most medical communities occupy different corners of the medical black box. The black box houses misunderstanding, misconception and considerable anxiety in the treatment of unfamiliar patient populations. Despite the commonality of black box occupation, there exists a wide gap between the disciplines of neurology and obstetrics. Neurologic disorders are reserved for neurologists. Pregnancy in most medical minds remains the exclusive area of obstetricians and a few family practice physicians. This type of specialism is adequate until neurologic problems coexist with pregnancy. It is then that members of two disciplines are required to leave their respective corners of the black box. Treatment of pregnant patients with neurologic disorders requires the two disciplines to meet, communicate and cooperate in patient care. This current work is intended to facilitate understanding and treatment in that area of the black box where neurology and obstetrics meet.

This work includes categories of neurologic problems that occur during pregnancy. The neurologic problems may be divided into three categories. The first category involves treatment of pre-existing neurologic problems during pregnancy; the chapters on headache, multiple sclerosis and epilepsy best fit into this category. The second category includes neurologic problems that are a direct consequence of pregnancy; the chapters on stroke, back pain and some peripheral nerve injuries are examples of this category. The discussions on treatment of infection, myasthenia gravis and peripheral nerve disorders are included in a third category; this category includes neurologic problems that require special treatment considerations during pregnancy and in the potentially pregnant patient. The three categories are covered by the authors in a concise informative manner.

This book will prove to be a resource for obstetricians, neurologists, students of both disciplines and other physicians who provide medical care to women of child-bearing age. The treatment of patients in this group must include consideration of the effect of pregnancy on the disorder, the effect of the disorder on pregnancy and potential effects of proposed therapies on the developing fetus. These considerations are not the exclusive concern of neurologists and obstetricians. The most common neurologic diagnoses are commonly managed by non-neurologists. Examples of these areas include headache, epilepsy, multiple sclerosis and the treatment of CNS infections. For that reason this book is a valuable resource for the care of women in many disciplines.

I would like to acknowledge my debt to the contributing authors for lending their expertise to this endeavor. I would also like to express my gratitude to Mr Jonathan Gregory and Mrs Pamela Lancaster from Parthenon Publishing for their encouragement and support.

Jaqueline M. Washington, MD

1

Migraine, pregnancy and lactation

S. D. Silberstein

INTRODUCTION

The International Headache Society (IHS)[1] divides headaches into two broad categories: primary and secondary headache disorders. Secondary headaches are attributed to another disorder, and can be caused by intracranial or extracranial structural abnormalities or by systemic or metabolic conditions. In primary headache disorders, the headache itself is the illness (Table 1). Primary headache disorders include migraine, tension-type headache (TTH) and cluster headache. Chronic daily headaches (CDH), a term in common use but not recognized by the IHS, may be due to chronic TTH, prolonged or transformed migraine, or hemicrania continua, and is often associated with abortive medication overuse[1].

Headache prevalence is age-dependent. Migraine prevalence peaks near age 40 and declines thereafter. With aging, there is not only a change in prevalence of the primary headache disorder, but also a shift to new or organic causes of headache[2].

The first step in establishing a headache diagnosis is a complete history, which should include the patient's age at headache onset; the location, severity and type of pain; the attack frequency (including any change in frequency); associated symptoms; precipitating and relieving factors; the patient's sleep habits; and the family history. A complete medication history should be taken to evaluate the doses, duration of use and effectiveness of previous headache medications, as well as to determine whether any medications that could exacerbate headaches are being used or overused[3]. This will serve only as a baseline, but will help with preconceptual counseling.

Migraine and TTH are primary headache disorders whose diagnosis is primarily clinical, with normal physical and neurologic examinations

Table 1 International Headache Society classification

Primary disorders
(1) Migraine
(2) Tension-type headache
(3) Cluster headache and chronic paroxysmal hemicrania
(4) Miscellaneous headaches unassociated with structural lesion
Secondary disorders
(5) Headache associated with head trauma
(6) Headache associated with vascular disorders
(7) Headache associated with non-vascular intracranial disorder
(8) Headache associated with substances or their withdrawal
(9) Headache associated with non-cephalic infection
(10) Headache associated with metabolic disorder
(11) Headache or facial pain associated with disorder of cranium, neck, eyes, ears, nose, sinuses, teeth, mouth or other facial or cranial structures
(12) Cranial neuralgias, nerve trunk pain and deafferentation pain

and a history that satisfies the IHS criteria[1]. However, conditions that mimic migraine may also occur during pregnancy[4]. New-onset migraine with aura can be due to a symptomatic disorder such as vasculitis, brain tumor or occipital arteriovenous malformation (AVM)[5]. Some disorders that produce headache, such as stroke, cerebral venous thrombosis, eclampsia and subarachnoid hemorrhage (SAH), occur more frequently during pregnancy. Sinusitis, meningitis and idiopathic intracranial hypertension can present as intractable headache[5]. SAH can present as a severe bout of acute-onset headache. These symptomatic conditions require neuroimaging and/or a lumbar puncture to diagnose them. Some disorders are more common or occur exclusively during pregnancy, and produce headache. These include stroke, cerebral venous thrombosis, eclampsia, SAH, pituitary tumor and choriocarcinoma[6,7]. Idiopathic intracranial hypertension does not occur more commonly than expected during pregnancy.

Investigation of headache, and migraine in particular, is controversial, and few guidelines exist. In fact, in a typical healthy migraineur, laboratory tests may not be necessary for diagnosis; some, however, are usually recommended prior to treatment. Even less is known about the need to investigate other types of headache. Systemic secondary causes of headache often cannot be diagnosed by physical examination; therefore, laboratory studies are performed to rule them out[5].

DIAGNOSTIC TESTING

Diagnostic testing functions to:

(1) Confirm the diagnosis;

(2) Exclude other causes of headache;

(3) Rule out comorbid and coexistent diseases that could complicate headache and its treatment;

(4) Establish a baseline for and exclude contraindications to drug treatment;

(5) Measure drug levels to determine absorption, patient compliance or medication overuse[8].

Lumbar puncture

Lumbar puncture is crucial in four distinct clinical situations:

(1) A 'first-or-worst' headache, with the suspicion of an intracranial infection or SAH;

(2) A severe, rapid-onset, recurrent headache;

(3) A progressive headache;

(4) A chronic intractable or atypical headache disorder[9]. If increased intracranial pressure is suspected, lumbar puncture should be performed after neuroimaging, except when meningitis is suspected, in which case it should not be delayed.

Neuroimaging

Head computerized tomography (CT) is relatively safe during pregnancy, and is the study of choice for head trauma and possible non-traumatic subarachnoid, subdural or intraparenchymal hemorrhage. For all other non-traumatic or non-hemorrhagic craniospinal pathology, magnetic resonance imaging (MRI) is preferred. Use MRI first to evaluate any suspected vascular pathology, but when necessary, angiography is reasonably safe in the pregnant patient (Table 2).

Indications for CT or MRI in headache investigation during pregnancy include: the first or worst headache of the patient's life, particularly if it is of abrupt onset (thunderclap headache); a change in the frequency, severity or clinical features of the headache attack; an abnormal neurologic examination; a progressive or new daily persistent

Table 2 Guidelines for neuroimaging the patient who is or may be pregnant. Adapted from reference 10

Determine the necessity and the potential risks of the procedure
If possible, perform the examination during the first 10 days postmenses, or if the patient is pregnant, delay the examination until the third trimester or preferably postpartum
Pick the procedure with the highest accuracy balanced by the lowest radiation
Use magnetic resonance imaging if possible
Avoid direct exposure to the abdomen and pelvis
Avoid contrast agents
Do not avoid radiologic testing purely for the sake of the pregnancy
If significant exposure is incurred by a pregnant patient, consult a radiation biologist
Consent forms are neither required nor recommended

headache; neurologic symptoms that do not meet the criteria of migraine with typical aura; persistent neurologic defects; definite electroencepalogram (EEG) evidence of a focal cerebral lesion; an orbital or skull bruit suggestive of AVM; and new comorbid partial (focal) seizures[5].

MIGRAINE

Migraine is an episodic headache disorder that may be preceded by a prodrome and initiated by an aura. In the past, migraine headaches were known as either classic migraine or common migraine, based on the presence or absence of an aura[4]. Common migraine is now called 'migraine without aura'. Classic migraine is now called 'migraine with aura'. Migraine with or without aura may be associated with premonitory phenomena that develop hours to days before the headache attack. Examples include hyper- or hypoactivity, depression, irritability, difficulty concentrating or food cravings, especially for chocolate[4].

Prevalence

Migraine occurs in 4% of children, 6% of men and 18% of women. Sixty-two per cent of migraineurs also have TTH[11]. Migraine usually begins in the first three decades of life, and prevalence peaks in the fifth decade[11]. The prognosis for migraine sufferers is good, since migraine prevalence decreases with increasing age[12]. Migraine in women is influenced by hormonal changes throughout the life cycle: menarche, menstruation, oral contraceptive use, pregnancy, menopause and hormone replacement therapy. Migraine can occur for the first time during pregnancy; pre-existing migraine may worsen, particularly during the first trimester; or the patient may become headache-free in later pregnancy. Some women have no change in their headache during pregnancy[13]. The true incidence of migraine in pregnancy is uncertain, and most reported cases have been of migraine with aura or prolonged aura. Migraine prevalence decreases with menopause, although the prevalence does not fall to premenarche levels.

Clinical features

Migraine diagnosis depends on the characteristics of the pain and associated features. A diagnosis of migraine without aura, according to IHS criteria (Table 3), requires the patient to have at least five headache attacks[1]. A diagnosis of migraine with aura (classic migraine) requires the patient to have at least two attacks with at least three characteristics listed in Table 4. If the aura lasts longer than 1 h but less than a week, the condition is called migraine with prolonged aura[1]. The migraine aura may occur without the headache, and migraine may remit or become transformed into CDH (with or without medication overuse).

Migraine aura occurs in about 20% of migraineurs. It usually develops over 5–20 min, lasts 20–30 min, and consists of focal neurologic symptoms (visual, sensory, motor or speech) that accompany the headache or occur up to an hour before it begins[14]. Visual symptoms are the

Table 3 Migraine without aura[1]

Diagnostic criteria

(A) At least five attacks fulfilling B–D

(B) Headache lasting 4–72 h (untreated or unsuccessfully treated)

(C) Headache has at least two of the following characteristics:
- (1) Unilateral location
- (2) Pulsating quality
- (3) Moderate or severe intensity (inhibits or prohibits daily activities)
- (4) Aggravation by walking stairs or similar routine physical activity

(D) During headache at least one of the following:
- (1) Nausea and/or vomiting
- (2) Photophobia and phonophobia

(E) No evidence of organic disease

Table 4 Migraine with aura[1]

Diagnostic criteria

(A) At least two attacks fulfilling B

(B) At least three of the following four characteristics:

(1) One or more fully reversible aura symptoms indicating focal cerebral cortical, brain stem dysfunction or both
(2) At least one aura symptom develops gradually over more than 4 min, or two or more symptoms occur in succession
(3) No aura symptom lasts more than 60 min. If more than one aura symptom is present, accepted duration is proportionally increased
(4) Headache follows aura with a free interval of less than 60 min. (It may also begin before or simultaneously with the aura)

(C) No evidence of organic disease

most common, and include scintillations (fluorescent flashes of light in the visual field), fortification spectra or teichopsia (alternating light and dark lines in the visual field), photopsia (flashing lights), positive scotomata (bright geometric lights in the visual field) and negative scotomata (blind spots that may move across the visual field). Sensory symptoms are less common and include numbness, tingling or paresthesias of the face or hand. Motor symptoms are usually hemiparetic, while language disturbances consist of difficulty speaking (aphasia) or understanding[15,16].

The headache of migraine can begin at any time during the day, usually developing gradually and subsiding after 4–72 h[17]. (A headache lasting longer than 72 h defines status migrainosus.) The pain is moderate to severe in intensity and usually described as throbbing or pulsating. It is usually unilateral, but may begin as, or become, bilateral[17]. Strictly unilateral headaches are not of concern since they occur in 20% of migraineurs. Accompanying symptoms are common: most patients are anorectic and have nausea; some vomit or have diarrhea. Photophobia and phonophobia cause patients to seek relief in a dark, quiet room to decrease sensory stimulation. Most patients have 1–4 attacks per month[16].

After the headache phase, some patients experience a postdrome, or recovery, phase that may last up to 24 h. Some patients feel tired, others feel alert, some feel depressed, others feel euphoric, some feel worn out while some feel refreshed. Some may complain of poor concentration, food intolerance or scalp tenderness[14].

Table 5 Tension-type headache[1]

Episodic tension-type headache

Diagnostic criteria

(A) At least ten previous headache episodes fulfilling criteria B–D listed below. Number of days with such headache < 180/year (< 15/month)

(B) Headache lasting from 30 min to 7 days

(C) At least two of the following pain characteristics:

(1) Pressing/tightening (non-pulsating) quality
(2) Mild or moderate intensity (may inhibit, but does not prohibit activities)
(3) Bilateral location
(4) No aggravation by walking stairs or similar routine physical activity

(D) Both of the following:

(1) No nausea or vomiting (anorexia may occur)
(2) Photophobia and phonophobia are absent, or one but not the other is present

Chronic tension-type headache

Diagnostic criteria

(A) Average headache frequency > 15 days/month (180 days/year) for > 6 months fulfilling criteria B–C

(B) At least two of the following pain characteristics:

(1) Pressing/tightening quality
(2) Mild or moderate severity (may inhibit but does not prohibit activities)
(3) Bilateral location
(4) No aggravation by walking stairs or similar routine physical activity

(C) Both of the following:

(1) No vomiting
(2) No more than one of the following: nausea, photophobia or phonophobia

Tension-type headache

TTH is the most common headache type, with a lifetime prevalence of 69% in men and 88% in women. TTH can begin at any age, but onset during adolescence or young adulthood is most common. The IHS criteria for TTH are listed in Table 5. The headache may be shorter or longer in duration than migraine. TTH is mild or moderate in intensity and has no accompanying autonomic symptoms. The cause of this common disorder is unknown, but it is not related to muscular tension (in fact, patients with migraine have more muscle tension than patients with TTH).

Table 6 Chronic daily headache[1]

Primary
Headache duration greater than 4 h
transformed (chronic) migraine (TM)
chronic tension-type headache (CTTH)
new daily persistent headache (NDPH)
hemicrania continua (HC)
Headache duration less than 4 h
cluster headache
chronic paroxysmal hemicrania
hypnic headache
idiopathic stabbing headache
Secondary
Post-traumatic headache (PTH)
Cervical spine disorders
Headache associated with vascular disorders (arteriovenous malformation, arteritis (including giant cell arteritis), dissection, subdural hematoma)
Headache associated with non-vascular intracranial disorders (intracranial hypertension, infection (EBV, HIV), neoplasm)
Other (temporomandibular joint disorder; sinus infection)

EBV, Epstein–Barr virus; HIV, human immunodeficiency virus

Acute TTH often responds to non-pharmacologic treatment. If the headache does not respond to this approach and medication is needed, many patients self-medicate with over-the-counter analgesics (aspirin, acetaminophen, ibuprofen, naproxen), with or without caffeine. Combination analgesics contain sedatives or caffeine and their use should be limited, as overuse may cause dependence. Narcotic analgesics and benzodiazepines should be avoided owing to their abuse potential. Overusing symptomatic medications, including tranquilizers and analgesics, can cause episodic TTH (ETTH) to convert to chronic TTH (CTTH)[18]. In women who are pregnant or attempting to become pregnant, the drugs should be used with the precautions outlined in the 'Headache treatment' section later in the chapter.

Chronic daily headache

CDH (Table 6) may be due to CTTH (Table 5) or transformed migraine, and is often associated with abortive medication overuse. It is important to determine the cause of the CDH so that the appropriate treatment can be chosen. When concurrent depression and medication dependence accompany CDH, treatment is difficult and detoxification may be required. This is particularly important for women who want to become pregnant. Under these circumstances, both the amounts and types of medicine used must be limited. Refractory rebound headaches

Table 7 Cluster headache[1]

(A)	At least five attacks fulfilling B–D
(B)	Severe unilateral orbital, supraorbital and/or temporal pain lasting 15–180 min untreated
(C)	Headache is associated with at least one of the following signs which have to be present on the pain side: (1) Conjunctival injection (2) Lacrimation (3) Nasal congestion (4) Rhinorrhea (5) Forehead and facial sweating (6) Miosis (7) Ptosis (8) Eyelid edema
(D)	Frequency of attacks: from one every other day to eight per day
(E)	No evidence of organic disease

may occur when aspirin, acetaminophen or opiate-containing analgesics are overused, or when analgesics are taken more frequently than 3 days per week, or ergotamine tartrate more often than 2 days per week. To avoid this situation, headache medication must be used within defined limits[18].

Cluster headache

Cluster headache prevalence is lower than that of migraine or TTH, with a rate of 0.01–0.24% in various populations. In contrast to migraine, prevalence is higher in men (70–90%) than in women (Table 7). Cluster headache can begin at any age: it most commonly begins in the late 20s, rarely in childhood, and occasionally (10%) in patients in their 60s[2,19]. The prognosis of cluster headaches is guarded; it is a chronic headache disorder that may last for the patient's entire life.

Episodic cluster features bouts that last from 1 week to a year with remission periods that last at least 14 days, whereas chronic cluster has either no remission periods or remissions that last less than 14 days. Cluster attacks may begin with slight discomfort that rapidly increases (within 15 min) to excruciating pain. The attacks often occur at the same time each day, and frequently awaken patients from sleep. Attacks generally last for 30–90 min, but may last up to 180 min and often occur once or twice a day. Patients may say, 'It's like a hot poker being driven into my eye'. Tearing occurs in most patients. Patients with cluster headaches should avoid alcohol and nitroglycerine.

DIFFERENTIAL DIAGNOSIS

A headache of sudden onset and extended duration may result from an SAH or an unruptured aneurysm. More benign causes of this condition include crash migraine and coital cephalalgia[5].

Thunderclap headache

Thunderclap headache is defined as the sudden onset of a severe headache that reaches maximum intensity within 1 min. Some further define it by the absence of an SAH. An acute neurologic event must be ruled out in all patients who present with severe, acute-onset headache, even though migraine can present in this manner.

Exertional and cough headaches

Transient, severe head pain upon coughing, sneezing, weight-lifting, bending, straining at stool or stooping defines exertional headache. MRI must be performed at the appropriate time to rule out hind-brain abnormalities, such as brain tumor (most commonly meningioma), Arnold–Chiari malformation, pineal cyst, basilar impression and acoustic neurinoma. If no abnormality is found, the diagnosis of benign cough headache may be made.

Other serious organic causes of headache

Several structural brain abnormalities can cause intense, bilateral headaches that last for minutes. Colloid cysts and other third ventricle masses may produce intermittent headaches with dizziness, blurred or double vision (some due to sixth nerve palsy), drop attacks and, rarely, sudden death.

Headache associated with mass lesions

Headache occurs at presentation in as many as 50% of patients with brain tumors, and develops in the course of the disease in 60% of them. Headache is partly dependent on tumor location: it is a rare initial symptom in patients with pituitary tumors, craniopharyngiomas or cerebellopontine angle tumors[20].

The postulated mechanisms of headache development include traction on pain-sensitive intracerebral vessels, transient herniation of hippocampal gyri, traction on cranial or cervical nerves or elevation of intracranial pressure. Although increased cerebrospinal fluid (CSF) pressure is not necessary for headache development, it clearly plays a role in a group of patients with central nervous system neoplasms[20].

In a modern series, 111 consecutive patients with primary (34%) or metastatic (66%) brain tumor were diagnosed by neuroimaging procedures[21]. Increased intracranial pressure was defined by the presence of papilledema, obstructive hydrocephalus, communicating hydrocephalus from leptomeningeal metastasis or a lumbar puncture opening pressure greater than 250 mm of CSF. Headache, present in 48% of both primary and metastatic tumors, was similar to TTH in 77% and to migraine in 9% of patients. Unlike true TTH, brain tumor headaches were worsened by bending in 32% of patients, and nausea or vomiting was present in 40%[21].

Most patients with increased intracranial pressure had a bilateral, frontal, aching headache; only 1% had a unilateral headache. The headache was constant in 61%. The pain was often severe, associated with nausea and vomiting, and resistant to common analgesics. Ataxia was present in 61%. In contrast, only 36% of patients with a supratentorial tumor without increased intracranial pressure had headache. These headaches were milder and more likely to be intermittent (however, they were constant in 20% of patients). Nausea, vomiting and ataxia were much less common[21].

There is a significant overlap between brain tumor headache and migraine and TTH. A headache of recent onset or a headache that has changed in character, particularly if the headache is severe or occurs with nausea or vomiting, or any neurologic sign or symptom that occurs with a headache and cannot be easily explained by the aura of migraine, requires a thorough evaluation. Morning or nocturnal headache associated with vomiting, and increased headache frequency, can be seen with both migraine and brain tumor. Brain tumor headache is more common in patients with a history of prior headache, increased intracranial pressure and large tumors with a midline shift[20].

Patients with brain abscesses, in contrast, often have a progressively severe, intractable headache. In a published clinical series, headache was present in 70–90% of patients who had a brain abscess[22]. The higher headache prevalence in abscess, compared to tumor, may be due to its faster evolution, the associated meningeal reaction and the occasional low-grade fever that may accompany an abscess.

Postpartum headache

Ponder[23] reviewed the differential diagnosis of postdural headache in the postpartum period. The two most frequently used methods for providing analgesia and anesthesia for labor and Cesarean section are spinal and epidural analgesia/anesthesia. One well-known complication is postdural puncture headache. Headaches in the parturient are usually attributed to a spinal anesthetic or an accidental dural puncture. After spinal anesthesia, non-postdural puncture headaches occur in 5–16% of patients. Headache occurs in 25% of parturients who have no neuroaxial anesthetic intervention. Pneumocephalus was a complication of epidural anesthesia with loss of resistance with 3–5 ml of air technique, even when there was no evidence of dural insult or difficult placement[24–26]. Pneumocephalus is characterized by an immediate to almost immediate sensation of back pain at the level of needle insertion, which then spreads rapidly cephalad to the posterior neck and on to the occipital and frontal areas. Mild to severe frontal, bifrontal, occipitofrontal, retro-orbital or generalized headache results from direct meningeal irritation. Maternal cortical vein thrombosis is an unusual complication of pregnancy, with the majority of episodes occurring within the first and third weeks postpartum[27]. Subdural hematoma is a rare complication of a spinal anesthetic, accidental dural puncture complicating an epidural anesthetic[28–32]. Subdural hematoma is due to the persistent leakage of CSF through the dural rent. Spontaneous subarachnoid hemorrhage, owing to aneurysms and arteriovenous malformations, occurs with an incidence of 1–5/10 000 pregnancies, which is higher than the incidence for the general population. The incidence of aseptic meningitis, injection of an irritant into the subarachnoid space, has decreased to near zero with modern techniques. Septic meningitis may occur as a result of a break in sterile technique or from contamination with an infectious agent present in blood or other tissue space. Postpartum headaches may be the harbinger of a serious medical event. Misdiagnosis of postdural puncture headache and resultant placement of an epidural blood patch can cloud and confuse further neurologic work-ups. Placement of an epidural blood patch in a parturient complaining of a headache that is a result of increased intracranial pressure can result in further exacerbation of symptoms, herniation or even death[28,33].

PREGNANCY AND MIGRAINE

Mechanisms

The relationship between migraine and sex hormones is well-known. Menarche, menstruation, oral contraceptive use, pregnancy, menopause and hormone replacement therapy affect migraine, in part by changing a woman's estrogen levels. Estrogen levels do not differ in non-pregnant women with or without menstrual migraine. Rising or sustained high estrogen levels have been proposed as the mechanism of migraine relief that often occurs during pregnancy; this mechanism, however, cannot explain the worsening or new appearance of migraine that sometimes occurs[34]. The rapid fall of estrogen levels may be responsible for menstrual and postpartum migraine. Women with a prior history of migraine are more likely to develop postpartum migraine[35].

Migraine relief during pregnancy is not dependent on adequate 'protective' levels of progesterone. Progesterone levels, measured near term, showed no statistical differences between women who did not have migraine relief during pregnancy and those who did, suggesting that migraine relief does not depend on the absolute blood level of progesterone[36].

The key to the genesis of migraine may be the intrinsic estrogen receptor sensitivity of the hypothalamic neurons. Although rising or sustained estrogen levels decrease headache in most women, these changes induce headache in some women[37].

Course of migraine during and after pregnancy

Approximately 60–70% of migraineurs will improve during pregnancy, while some women who have not had migraine will experience their first migraine headache. Case reports of migraine that occur for the first time during pregnancy emphasize the presence of focal neurologic symptoms (migraine with aura), probably because patients with these dramatic presentations are more likely to be referred to a neurologist. Wright and Patel[38] presented a series of ten women with headache and focal neurologic symptoms (visual or sensory aura, dysphasia, weakness or a combination of these symptoms); two presented in the first trimester, six in the third trimester and two postpartum. Massey[39] reported a 19-year-old woman who, in her 27th week of pregnancy, developed two episodes (24 h apart) of anomia, blurred vision and right arm, face and mouth numbness, followed by a pounding bifrontal headache with photophobia.

Chancellor and Wroe[34] presented a series of nine women who developed migraine for the first time while pregnant. One woman had migraine without aura; eight had migraine with aura. Two women developed migraine in the first trimester of pregnancy, two in the second trimester and five in the third. These women were referred for neurologic consultation because of focal neurologic symptoms. Four patients developed complications: two had pre-eclampsia, one a threatened abortion and two (one of whom had pre-eclampsia) had premature deliveries.

We[40] reported a 27-year-old woman with no family or personal history of migraine who presented with a headache associated with unilateral paresthesias and blurred vision. This was her first attack of migraine with aura, and led to the diagnosis of her pregnancy.

Lance and Anthony[41] retrospectively studied 120 migraineurs who had borne children. Migraine improved in 58% of these women, while 42% worsened or had no change in their migraine. Sixty-four per cent of women with menstrual migraine had relief during pregnancy, compared to 48% of those who had non-menstrual migraine. These authors did not look at migraine incidence during pregnancy.

Callaghan[42] interviewed 200 women between the ages of 16 and 48 in the department of obstetrics at an Irish hospital. Only eight women had migraine before their pregnancy; of these, four improved. The prevalence of migraine among women is 19%[37]. It is even higher among fertile women. Callaghan's 4% prevalence of pre-existing migraine (8/200) is extraordinarily low, and makes his statistics suspect. Thirty-three of the 200 patients developed migraine during pregnancy, new attacks occurring during each trimester (16 during the first, nine during the second and eight during the third trimester).

Callaghan's[42] finding that migraine prevalence during pregnancy is much higher than migraine prevalence prior to pregnancy prompted Somerville[43] to study an antenatal population of 200 women in Australia in the early 1970s. Thirty-eight had migraine, 31 had a prior history of migraine and seven developed migraine while pregnant (five women in the first trimester, one in the second trimester and one in the third trimester). Seventy-seven per cent of women with pre-existing migraine improved during their pregnancy. Somerville did not distinguish between migraine with and without aura.

Bousser's group[44] interviewed 703 patients shortly after delivery in an attempt to study the relationship between IHS-defined migraine[1] and pregnancy. One hundred and sixteen women (147 pregnancies) fulfilled the IHS criteria for migraine. Pre-existing migraine improved or disappeared in 102/131 pregnancies (77.9%), worsened in ten (7.6%), was unchanged in 11 (8.4%) and was variable in eight (6.1%). Migraine appeared for the first time in 16 women. Disappearance or improvement did not differ significantly in migraine with or without aura, but worsening was much more common in migraine with aura. Improvement was more frequent in women with menstrual migraine. No significant difference was found in the evolution of migraine in any of the three trimesters of pregnancy.

Granella and colleagues[45] retrospectively analyzed 1300 migraineurs attending a headache clinic in Italy: complete remission occurred in 17.4%; 49.2% had significant improvement; and only 3.5% worsened. Women whose migraine started with menarche had a higher remission rate (36.4% vs. 13.99) than women whose headaches began at other times. Migraine began during pregnancy in 1.3% of the patients and postpartum in 4.5%.

Rasmussen[46] evaluated 1000 women in a cross-sectional epidemiologic study. Eighty migraineurs in the group had been pregnant. Of these, 48% had no change, 49% had disappearance or significant improvement in their headache and only 4% worsened.

Chen and Leviton[47] analyzed the data from the Prospective Collaborative Perinatal Project of 55 000 pregnant women in the USA. Only 2% of these women had self-reported migraine, an under-ascertainment of true migraine prevalence perhaps because only severe cases were identified. Of those analyzable (484), 17% had a complete remission and another 62% showed some improvement with pregnancy. No correlation to menstrual migraine was attempted.

Scharff and colleagues[48] recruited 30 women who were more than 10 weeks pregnant. They reported a non-significant decrease in all headache types including migraine and TTH, more so for the primiparous women.

Maggioni and associates[49] evaluated 428 women 3 days postpartum. Eighty-one had migraine without aura and 12 had migraine with aura. One new case of migraine without aura began during pregnancy. Of the migraineurs, 86% had at least a 50% decrease in attack frequency, usually after the first trimester.

Granella and co-workers[50] evaluated the relationship between migraine with aura and the milestones of reproductive life. A retrospective case–control study was carried out of 100 women affected by migraine with typical aura (cases) and 200 age-matched women with migraine without aura (controls). Premenstrual syndrome was found to be much more common among the patients with migraine with aura (odds ratio (OR) 6.0, 95% confidence interval (CI) 3.1–11.6). Menstrually triggered migraine was more frequently encountered among migraine without aura than migraine with aura patients (migraine with aura 15.0%, migraine without aura 53.5%; OR 0.1, CI 0.1–0.3). In both forms of migraine, pregnancy had a favorable effect; however, a lower percentage of migraine with aura (43.6%) than migraine without aura patients (76.8%; OR 0.2, CI 0.1–0.5) showed improvement or remission.

Sances and colleagues[51] prospectively investigated the course of migraine during pregnancy and postpartum, in consecutive pregnant women attending an obstetrics and gynecology department for a routine first-trimester antenatal check-up. Forty-nine migraineurs, two with migraine with aura and 47 with migraine without aura, who had experienced at least one attack during the 3 months preceding pregnancy were identified, enrolled in the study and given a headache diary. Follow-up examinations were performed at the end of the second and third trimesters and 1 month after delivery. Migraine improved in 46.8% of the 47 migraine without aura sufferers during the first trimester, in 83.0% during the second and in 87.2% during the third, while complete remission was attained by 10.6%, 53.2% and 78.7% of the women, respectively. Risk factors for lack of improvement in the second trimester included menstrually related migraine (a lack of headache improvement in the first and third trimesters), second-trimester hyperemesis and a pathological pregnancy course. At variance with other authors, and quite surprisingly, Sances and colleagues found that the occurrence of menstrually related migraine prior to pregnancy constituted a risk factor for a lack of improvement in both the first and the third trimesters. An explanation of the phenomenon may lie in their definition of menstrually related migraine, which included not only migraine occurring solely during menses, but also migraine occurring during and outside menses.

Wainscott and Volans[52] found that the incidence of miscarriage, toxemia, congenital anomalies and stillbirth was not increased in a sample of 777 migraine sufferers compared with the national averages or controls. However, in Chancellor's small series, four of nine patients developed complications, including pre-eclampsia in two. Again, this may be due to selection artifact. Olesen and colleagues[53] recently found that the odds ratio for having a newborn with a low birth weight was increased (OR 3.0, 95% CI 1.3–7.0) for all migraine patients who delivered at term (n = 115) compared with the outcome of healthy pregnancies.

Stein[35] prospectively followed 71 randomly selected women during their first postpartum week. Postnatal headache (PNH) occurred in 39%. It was most frequent on days 3–6 postpartum, and was associated with a past history or a family history of migraine. PNH, while less severe than the patients' typical migraine, was bifrontal, prolonged and associated with photophobia, nausea and anorexia.

MacArthur and associates[54] investigated 11 701 women who gave birth in one hospital in Birmingham between 1978 and 1985. Follow-up information was obtained by postal questionnaire. By 3 months postpartum, newly occurring frequent headache occurred in 3.6% of the women and migraine in 1.4%. The definition of migraine was not stated. Two of Wright and Patel's[38] cases of focal neurologic migraine presented postpartum. Both had a history of migraine with aura. Migraine frequently restarts in the postpartum period and can begin *de novo*.

Sances and colleagues[51] found that migraine recurred during the first week after childbirth in 34.0% of the women and during the first month in 53.3%. Bottle-feeding was found to be associated with migraine recurrence.

Most women with migraine improve during pregnancy, women without aura more commonly than women with aura. Some women have their first attack during pregnancy. Migraine often recurs postpartum and can begin for the first time in general. Despite drug use, migraineurs do not differ from non-migraineurs in miscarriages, toxemia, congenital anomalies or stillbirth.

DRUGS AND PREGNANCY

Overview

It used to be believed that the placenta served as a barrier that protected the fetus from drugs and toxins[55]. However, recognition of the teratogenicity of aminopterin and thalidomide, and the rubella epidemic of 1963–64, changed this perception and resulted in extremely conservative drug use during pregnancy[8]. In 1977 the Food and Drug Administration (FDA) developed a policy against phase I and early phase II testing in pregnant women or in women of child-bearing potential, and many practitioners now avoid drug treatment in pregnancy even when it is indicated. The FDA has tested over 3000 drugs, and only 20 are known human teratogens. There is insufficient knowledge about birth defect risks from drug exposure, despite the fact that 67% of women take drugs during pregnancy and 50% take them during the first trimester[56].

Most drugs cross the placenta and have the potential to affect the fetus adversely, and, although studies have not absolutely established the safety of any medication during pregnancy, some are believed to be relatively safe.

A negative pregnancy test is often a condition of enrollment in a study, while postenrollment pregnancy can lead to termination of participation. This poses a problem for pregnant women who are sick and in need of treatment. If a drug has not been tested in pregnant women during the research phase, information is lacking about the safety and efficacy of the drug for the women as well as the fetus[57]. The Institute of Medicine Committee on Research in Women made the controversial recommendation that pregnant and lactating women be considered eligible for enrollment in clinical studies on a routine basis[57].

With more women of child-bearing age participating in clinical trials, more information will be gained about the risks of birth defects, but uncertainty will still persist. However, if the medication is associated with a very high level of birth defects (e.g. thalidomide), very few exposures need to be followed to detect this risk; if the medication is associated with a slight increase in the overall occurrence of birth defects, approximately 300 exposed pregnancies need to be followed to detect a doubling of risk; and if the medication is associated with a rare increase of a specific defect (e.g. 1/1000), approximately 10 000 exposed pregnancies need to be followed to detect a doubling of risk[58].

Epidemiology

The World Health Organization completed an international survey of 14 778 pregnant women on prescription drug utilization during pregnancy. Eighty-six per cent of the subjects took medication, each receiving an average of 2.9 prescriptions. Of a total of 37 309 prescriptions, 73% were given by obstetricians, 12% by general practitioners and 5% by midwives[59]. In a survey of pregnant women at Parkland Memorial Hospital in Dallas, 40% took some type of medication other than iron or vitamin supplements and up to 20% used an illicit drug or alcohol[60]. The National Hospital Discharge Survey found that there was a 576% increase in discharges of drug-using parturient women and a 456% increase in discharges of drug-affected newborns in the USA between 1979 and 1990.

Adverse effects

Adverse drug effects depend on the dose and route of administration, concomitant exposures and timing of the exposure relative to the period of development (i.e. the preimplantation period, embryogenesis and fetal development). The preimplantation period lasts from conception to 1 week postconception, during which time the conceptus is relatively protected from drugs[60]. Embryogenesis is the time of organogenesis, which occurs from the time of implantation to 60 days postconception[60]. Most congenital malformations arise during this time. Placental transport is not well established until the fifth week after conception. This protects the embryo from maternal drugs. The final phase, fetal development, follows embryogenesis. The fetus grows mainly in size, although structural changes such as neuronal arrangement also occur. Malformations can develop at this time in normally formed organs owing to their necrosis and reabsorption[60].

Death to the conceptus, teratogenicity, fetal growth abnormalities, perinatal effects, postnatal developmental abnormalities, delayed oncogenesis and functional and behavioral changes can result from drugs or other agents (Table 8)[61]. According to the Perinatal Collaborative Project, a prospective and concurrent epidemiologic study of more than 50 000 pregnancies, many drugs have little or no human teratogenic risk[61].

Spontaneous abortion

Nearly half of early pregnancies abort spontaneously, most due to chromosomal abnormalities. Prior to the time of organogenesis, exposure to a potential teratogen or toxic drug has an all-or-none effect. Exposure around the time of conception or implantation may kill the conceptus,

Table 8 Definitions and drug effects

Spontaneous abortion	death of the conceptus. Most due to chromosomal abnormality
Embryotoxicity	the ability of drugs to kill the developing embryo
Congenital anomalies	deviation from normal morphology or function
Teratogenicity	the ability of an exogenous agent to produce a permanent abnormality of structure or function in an organism exposed during embryogenesis or fetal life
Fetal effects	growth restriction, abnormal histogenesis (also congenital abnormalities and fetal death). The main outcome of fetal drug toxicity during the second and third trimesters of pregnancy
Perinatal effects	effects on uterine contraction, neonatal withdrawal or hemostasis
Postnatal effects	drugs may have delayed long-term effects: delayed oncogenesis, and functional and behavioral abnormalities

but if the pregnancy continues, there is no increased risk of congenital anomalies[62].

Developmental defects

Developmental defects may result from genetic or environmental causes, or from interactions between them. Teratogenic drug effects are generally visible anatomic malformations; they are defined as the production of a permanent alteration of an organ's structure or function due to intrauterine exposure. These effects are dose- and time-related, with the fetus at greatest risk during the first trimester of pregnancy. Drug exposure accounts for only 2–3% of birth defects: approximately 25% are genetic and the causes of the remainder are unknown[62]. The incidence of major malformations either incompatible with survival or requiring major surgery is approximately 2–3% in the general population. If all minor malformations are included (ear tags or extra digits), the rate may be as high as 7–10%. The risk of malformation after drug exposure must be compared with this background rate.

The classic teratogenic period in the human is a critical 6 weeks, lasting from approximately 31 days to 10 weeks from the last menstrual period. A teratogenic effect depends on timing of the exposure as well as nature of the teratogen. Exposure early in pregnancy, when the heart and central nervous system are forming, may result in an anomaly such as congenital heart disease or neural tube defect, while later exposure may result in malformation of the palate or ear[62]. Once the teratogenic period has passed, the major risk of congenital anomaly is gone, but other abnormalities can occur. These include fetal effects, neonatal effects and postnatal effects.

Fetal effects

Fetal effects include damage to normally formed organs, damage to systems undergoing histogenesis, growth restriction or fetal death. Growth restriction is the most common of these.

Neonatal and postnatal effects

Certain drugs are associated with adverse neonatal effects, such as drug withdrawal and neonatal hypoglycemia, or adverse maternal effects, such as hemostasis and uterine contracture disorders. Chronic exposure to psychoactive medications, such as alcohol, during the second and third trimesters, may cause mental retardation, which may not be recognized until later in life[62]. Developmental delay and long-term cognitive dysfunction have been reported in children born to mothers who took antiepileptic drugs (AEDs) during pregnancy.

Delayed oncogenesis

Exposure to diethylstilbestrol as late as 20 weeks' gestation may cause reproductive organ anomalies that are not recognized until after puberty.

Drug risk categories

The FDA lists five categories of labeling for drug use in pregnancy (Table 9)[56,67–70]. These categories are intended to provide therapeutic guidance, weighing the risks as well as the benefits of the drug. Although this system is an improvement over previous labeling, it is still

Table 9 Food and Drug Administration risk categories

Category A	controlled human studies show no risk
Category B	no evidence of risk in humans, but there are no controlled human studies
Category C	risk to humans has not been ruled out
Category D	positive evidence of risk to humans from human and/or animal studies
Category X	contraindicated in pregnancy

Table 10 TERIS (an automated teratogen information resource) risk rating with equivalent Food and Drug Administration ratings in parentheses

N	none (A)
N-Min	none–minimal (A)
Min	minimal (B)
Min-S	minimal–small (D)
S	small ( )
S-Mod	small–moderate ( )
Mod	moderate ( )
H	high (X)
U	undetermined (C)

not ideal. The classification is often not changed when new data become available. Combined oral contraceptives were previously classified as category X, despite there being no evidence of increased risk or teratogenicity[55]. Tricyclic antidepressants are still classified as category D, even though the evidence suggests them to be safe[55]. An alternative rating system is TERIS, an automated teratogen information resource wherein the rating for each drug or agent is based on a consensus of expert opinion and the literature (Table 10)[64]. It was designed to assess the teratogenic risk to the fetus from a drug exposure. The FDA categories have little, if any, correlation to the TERIS teratogenic risk. This discrepancy results in part because the FDA categories were designed to provide therapeutic guidance and the TERIS ratings are useful for estimating the teratogenic risks of a drug, and not vice versa[65].

Prevention

A woman's risk of having a child with a neural tube defect is associated with early-pregnancy red cell folate levels in a continuous dose–response relationship[66]. Low serum and red blood cell folate levels are associated with spontaneous abortion and fetal malformations in animals and in humans[56,67–70]. Treatment with some drugs, including carbamazepine and barbiturates, can impair folate absorption. Valproic acid does not produce folate deficiency, but it may interfere with the production of folinic acid by inhibiting glutamate formyl transferase[71]. The current guidelines suggest increasing folic acid intake by 4 mg, which would result in a 48% reduction in neural tube defects[66].

Maternal physiology

Profound structural and physiologic changes occur during pregnancy[72]. The uterus rapidly increases in size, transformed from an almost-solid structure weighing 70 g into a relatively thin-walled, muscular organ large enough to accommodate the fetus, placenta and amniotic fluid[73]. Uterine growth depends on estrogen and, to a lesser extent, progesterone, during the first few months of pregnancy. After 12 weeks, growth results from the pressure exerted by the expanding products of conception. Cell and tissue growth is dependent on increased synthesis of polyamines (including spermidine and spermine and their immediate precursor, putrescine)[73].

Metabolic changes occur in response to the rapidly growing fetus and placenta. Weight gain, due to the increase in the uterus and its contents, the breasts, the blood volume and the extravascular extracellular fluid, averages about 11 kg, with about 1 kg occurring during the first trimester[73]. Water retention (about 6.5 l by term) is a normal occurrence, mediated in part by a fall in plasma osmolality of 10 mosmol/kg, owing to a resetting of the osmoreceptor. The fetus, placenta and amniotic fluid contain about 3.5 l of water. Another 3.0 l of water results from increased maternal blood volume and the increase in uterine and breast size. Near term, blood volume is about 45% above baseline. Weight loss during the first 10 days postpartum averages about 2 kg[73].

While pregnancy is potentially diabetogenic, in healthy pregnant women the fasting plasma glucose concentration may fall owing to increased plasma insulin levels. Progesterone, when administered to a non-pregnant adult in an amount similar to that produced during pregnancy, results in an increased basal insulin concentration and response to an oral glucose challenge similar to that of a normal pregnant woman. Additionally, estradiol induces hyperinsulinism in both control and ovariectomized rats[73].

Lipid, lipoprotein and apolipoprotein plasma concentrations increase during pregnancy. There is a positive correlation between lipid concentrations and levels of estradiol, progesterone and human placental lactogen.

The kidneys barely increase in size during pregnancy[74]. Early in pregnancy, at the beginning of the second trimester, the glomerular filtration rate and renal plasma flow increase by about 50%[75,76]. The elevated glomerular filtration rate persists to term, whereas the renal plasma flow decreases during late pregnancy[76]. The human liver does not increase in size during pregnancy, and we are not certain whether or not hepatic blood flow increases.

The profound physiologic changes that occur during pregnancy can alter drug pharmacokinetics: plasma volume increases by half, cardiac output increases by 30–50% and renal plasma flow and glomerular filtration rate increase by 40–50%. Serum albumin decreases by 20–30%, resulting in decreased drug binding and increased drug clearance. Increased extracellular fluid and adipose tissue increases the volume of drug distribution. Drug metabolism may also be increased, modulated in part by the high concentration of sex hormones[77].

Seizure frequency can increase during pregnancy owing to changes in AED concentration. Total concentrations of carbamazepine, phenytoin, phenobarbital and valproic acid fall as a result of decreased plasma protein binding, while free or unbound drug concentrations of only phenobarbital fall significantly. Valproate free concentrations actually increase by 25% by delivery[78].

The placenta is a lipid membrane barrier that separates the maternal and fetal circulation. Most drugs cross this barrier by simple diffusion. The rate of transfer is dependent on the drug's molecular size, lipid solubility and protein binding. Drugs with a very high molecular weight, such as heparin, do not cross the placenta easily, while drugs with a low molecular weight (< 6000 Da) cross it easily. Most drugs have steady-state levels at or near maternal levels, although some drugs may be trapped, with fetal levels 2–3 times maternal levels[79,80].

HEADACHE TREATMENT

The major concerns in management of the pregnant patient are the effects of both medication and disease on the fetus. Because of the possible risk of injury to the fetus, medication use should be limited; however, it is not contraindicated during pregnancy[56,81]. Since migraine usually improves after the first trimester, many women can manage their headaches with this reassurance and non-pharmacologic means of coping, such as ice, massage and biofeedback[56,82]. Some women, however, will continue to have severe, intractable headaches, sometimes associated with nausea, vomiting and possible dehydration. Not only are these conditions disruptive to the patient, they may pose a risk to the fetus that is greater than the potential risk of the medications used to treat the pregnant patient[81,82].

Symptomatic treatment, designed to reduce the severity and duration of symptoms, is used to treat an acute headache attack (Tables 11–16). Individual attacks should be treated with rest, reassurance and ice packs. For headaches that do not respond to non-pharmacologic treatment, symptomatic drugs are indicated. The non-steroidal anti-inflammatory drugs (NSAIDs), acetaminophen (alone or with codeine), codeine alone or other opioids can be used during pregnancy[55]. Aspirin in low intermittent doses is not a significant teratogenic risk, although large doses, especially if given near term, may be associated with maternal and fetal bleeding. Aspirin use should probably be reserved unless there is a definite therapeutic need for it (other than headache). In general, NSAIDs may be safely taken for pain during the first trimester of pregnancy. However, their use should be limited

Table 11 Ergots and serotonin agonists

	Fetal risk		
	FDA	*TERIS*	*Breast-feeding*
Ergots			
Ergotamine	X	Min	contraindicated
Dihydroergotamine	X	U	contraindicated
Methylergonovine	C	U	caution
Methysergide	X	U	caution
Triptans			
Sumatriptan	C	U	caution
Naratriptan	C	U	caution
Rizatriptan	C	U	caution
Zolmitriptan	C	U	caution

FDA, Food and Drug Administration; TERIS, automated teratogen information resource

Table 12 Analgesics

	Fetal risk		
	FDA	*TERIS*	*Breast-feeding*
Simple analgesics			
Aspirin	C*	N-Min	caution
Acetaminophen	B	N	compatible
Caffeine	B	N-min	compatible
NSAIDs			
Fenoprofen	B*	U	compatible
Ibuprofen`	B*	N-Min	compatible
Indomethacin	B*	N	compatible
Ketorolac	C*	U	caution
Meclofenamate	B*	U	compatible
Naproxen	B*	U	compatible
Sulindac	B*	U	compatible
Tolmetin	C*	U	caution

*D if third trimester; NSAIDs, non-steroidal anti-inflammatory drugs; FDA, Food and Drug Administration; TERIS, automated teratogen information resource

Table 13 Opioids

	Fetal risk		
	FDA	*TERIS*	*Breast-feeding*
Butorphanol	B*	N-Min	compatible
Codeine	C*	N-Min	compatible
Hydromorphone	B*	N-Min	compatible
Meperidine	B*	N-Min	compatible
Methadone	B*	N-Min	compatible
Morphine	B*	N-Min	compatible
Propoxyphene	C*	N-Min	compatible

*D if prolonged or at term; FDA, Food and Drug Administration; TERIS, automated teratogen information resource

Table 14 Corticosteroids

	Fetal risk		
	FDA	*TERIS*	*Breast-feeding*
Cortisone	D	N-Min	compatible
Dexamethasone	C	N-Min	compatible
Prednisone	B	N-Min	compatible
Triamcinolone	C	N-Min	compatible

FDA, Food and Drug Administration; TERIS, automated teratogen information resource

during later pregnancy, as some NSAIDs may constrict or close the fetal ductus arteriosus[55]. Byron[83] believes that the most potent inhibitors of prostaglandin synthesis, such as salicylates and indomethacin, should be avoided throughout pregnancy if possible, and certainly during the last trimester. Barbiturate and benzodiazepine use should be limited. Ergotamine, dihydroergotamine (DHE) and sumatriptan should be avoided[56,82].

The associated symptoms of migraine, such as nausea and vomiting, can be as disabling as the headache pain itself. In addition, some medications that are used to treat migraine can produce nausea. Metoclopramide, which decreases the gastric atony seen with migraine and enhances the absorption of coadministered medications, is extremely useful in migraine treatment[8]. Mild nausea can be treated with phosphorylated carbohydrate solution (emetrol) or doxylamine succinate and vitamin B_6 (pyridoxine)[8,55]. More severe nausea may

Table 15 Neuroleptics/antiemetics

	Fetal risk		
	FDA	*TERIS*	*Breast-feeding*
Other			
Emetrol	B	U	compatible
Doxylamine and vitamin B_6	B	N	NA
Trimethobenzamide	C	N-Min	NA
Neuroleptics			
Phenothiazines			
chlorpromazine	C	N-Min	concern
prochlorperazine	C	N	compatible
promethazine	C	N	NA
promazine	C	U	NA
Butyrophenones			
droperidol	C	U	unknown
haloperidol	C	N-Min	concern
Thioxanthenes			
thiothixene	C	U	NA
Other			
metoclopramide	B	N-Min	concern

FDA, Food and Drug Administration; TERIS, automated teratogen information resource; NA, not available

require the use of injections or suppositories. Trimethobenzamide, chlorpromazine, prochlorperazine and promethazine are available orally, parenterally and as a suppository, and can all be used safely. We frequently use promethazine and prochlorperazine suppositories. Corticosteroids can be utilized occasionally. Some use prednisone in preference to dexamethasone (which crosses the placenta more readily). Domperidone is an antiemetic used outside the USA. In the UK[84] its use is not advised during pregnancy, because of variable embryotoxic effects in animal tests. In France, in contrast, the product summary indicates no teratogenicity in animals or humans. Minimal amounts are transferred in breast milk.

Acute treatment

Severe acute attacks of migraine should be treated aggressively[81,85]. We start intravenous (IV) fluids for hydration and then use

Table 16 Sedatives/hypnotics/antihistamines

	Fetal risk		
	FDA	*TERIS*	*Breast-feeding*
Antihistamines			
Cyclizine	B	U	NA
Cyproheptadine	B	U	contraindicated
Dimenhydrinate	B	U	NA
Meclizine	B	N-Min	NA
Barbiturates			
Butalbital	C	N-Min	caution
Phenobarbital	D	N-Min	caution
Benzodiazepam			
Chlordiazepoxide	D	N-min	concern
Clonazepam	D	U	concern
Diazepam	D	N-Min	concern
Lorazepam	D	U	concern
Other			
Zolpidem	B	U	not recommended

FDA, Food and Drug Administration; TERIS, automated teratogen information resource; NA, not available

prochlorperazine 10 mg IV to control both nausea and head pain. IV opioids or IV corticosteroids can supplement this. This is an extremely effective way of handling status migrainosus during pregnancy.

Eldridge and colleagues[86] recently reviewed the Glaxo-Wellcome pregnancy registries (observational, case-registration and follow-up studies designed to detect evidence of teratogenicity associated with specific medications). After prenatal exposure to the registry medication, pregnancies are registered prospectively, through voluntary reports by health-care providers. The following data show results from the prospective first-trimester exposures registered since the establishment of each registry. The published risk of birth defects in the general population range is 3–5%, and the risk in women with epilepsy is 6–9%. The proportion of outcomes with birth defects is, in the sumatriptan (migraine medication) pregnancy registry (1996 – October 1998), 7/183 (3.8%; 95% CI 1.7–8.0%). The naratriptan registry has insufficient data for analysis. None of the registries has provided a risk estimate exceeding that expected in the disorder treated, and no pattern of defects has been observed. Whereas information from the larger registries is reassuring regarding risk, these studies cannot rule out possible small excess risks from use of these drugs in pregnancy.

Some 2.5% of fertile Danish women use sumatriptan, and continue to use it during pregnancy. Olesen and colleagues[53] analyzed data from the Pharmacoepidemiological Prescription Database of North Jutland county. All women who had given birth in the county of North Jutland from 1991 to 1996 were linked to the Danish Medical Birth Registry. Women exposed to sumatriptan during pregnancy were identified (n = 34), and using logistic regression models their pregnancy outcome was compared with two groups of pregnant women: healthy women (n = 15 955) and migraine controls (n = 89), defined as migraine patients who did not redeem prescriptions for migraine treatment during pregnancy. The risk of preterm delivery was elevated among women exposed to sumatriptan compared with migraine controls (OR 6.3, 95% CI 1.2–32.0) and healthy women (OR 3.3, 95% CI 1.3–8.5). The odds ratio for having a newborn with a low birth weight was increased (OR 3.0, 95% CI 1.3–7.0) for all migraine patients who delivered at term (n = 115), compared with the outcome of healthy pregnancies.

Källén and Lygner[87] evaluated delivery outcome in women who used drugs for migraine during pregnancy with special reference to sumatriptan. Using the Swedish Medical Birth Registry, which contains information on drug use reported by women at the first antenatal visit, 912 infants (born in 905 deliveries) whose mothers had used drugs for migraine were identified, the majority of whom (n = 658) had used sumatriptan. These women differed from the general population of women who had delivered by being older and more often of first parity, but they had similar smoking habits. Slightly more often, the infants were preterm, and they had a birth weight less than 2500 g; neither of these effects were statistically significant. There seemed to be no difference between infants exposed to sumatriptan and those exposed to other drugs used for migraine. No increase in the rate of congenital malformations was seen. In this study the use of sumatriptan in early pregnancy did not result in a large increase in teratogenic risk, but results do not rule out the possibility of a moderate increase in risk for a specific birth defect. Among the 16 infants with major malformations, nine were exposed to sumatriptan; 1.3% of infants exposed to sumatriptan and 2.8% of infants exposed to other drugs for migraine, but not to sumatriptan, had such malformations (p = 0.14).

Preventive treatment

Increased frequency and severity of migraine associated with nausea and vomiting may justify the use of daily prophylactic (preventive) med-

Table 17 Anticonvulsants

	Fetal risk		
	FDA	*TERIS*	*Breast-feeding*
Carbamazepine	C	S	compatible
Gabapentin	C	U	uncertain
Lamotrigine	C	U	not recommended
Phenobarbital	D	Min-S	compatible
Phenytoin	D	S-Mod	compatible
Primidone	D	S-Mod	caution
Topiramate	C	U	uncertain
Valproic acid	D	S-Mod	compatible
Vigabatrin		U	uncertain

FDA, Food and Drug Administration; TERIS, automated teratogen information resource

ication. This treatment option should be a last resort, and used only with the consent of the patient and her partner after the risks have been completely explained. Preventive therapy is designed to reduce the frequency and severity of headache attacks. Consider prophylaxis when patients experience at least three or four prolonged, severe attacks per month that are particularly incapacitating or unresponsive to symptomatic therapy and may result in dehydration and fetal distress[13,82]. β-Adrenergic blockers such as propranolol have been used under these circumstances, although adverse effects, including intrauterine growth restriction, have been reported[8,55]. If the migraine is so severe that drug treatment is essential, the patient should be told of the risks posed by all the drugs that are used (Tables 17–19)[13]. If the patient has a coexistent illness that requires treatment, pick one drug that will treat both disorders. For example, propranolol[55] can be used to treat hypertension and migraine, while fluoxetine can be used to treat comorbid depression.

Drug exposure

If a woman inadvertently takes a drug while she is pregnant or becomes pregnant while taking a drug, determine the dose, timing and duration of the exposure(s). Ascertain the patient's past and present state of

Table 18 Antidepressants

	Fetal risk		
	FDA	*TERIS*	*Breast-feeding*
Tricyclics			
Amitriptyline	D	N-Min	concern
Amoxapine	C	U	concern
Desipramine	C	U	concern
Doxepin	C	U	concern
Imipramine	D	N-Min	concern
Nortriptyline	D	U	concern
Protriptyline	C	U	concern
SSRIs			
Fluoxetine	B	N	caution
Paroxetine	C	U	concern?
Sertraline	B	U	concern?
MAOIs			
Phenelzine	C	U	concern
Others			
Bupropion	B	U	concern

SSRI, selective serotonin reuptake inhibitor; MAOI, monoamine oxidase inhibitor; FDA, Food and Drug Administration; TERIS, automated teratogen information resource

health, and the presence of mental retardation or chromosomal abnormalities in the family. Using a reliable source of information (such as TERIS), determine whether the drug is a known teratogen (although for many drugs this is not possible)[59,60,62,64].

If the drug is teratogenic or the risk is unknown, have the obstetrician confirm the gestational age by ultrasound. If the exposure occurred during embryogenesis, then high-resolution ultrasound can be performed to determine whether damage to specific organ systems or structures has occurred. If the high-resolution ultrasound is normal, it is reasonable to reassure the patient that the gross fetal structure is normal (within the 90% sensitivity of the study)[60]. However, fetal ultrasound cannot exclude minor anomalies or guarantee the birth of a normal child. Delays in achieving developmental milestones, including cognitive development, are potential risks that cannot be predicted or diagnosed prenatally. Have the obstetrician discuss the results of these studies with the mother and the significant other; formal prenatal counseling may be helpful in uncertain cases[60].

Table 19 Antihypertensives

	Fetal risk		
	FDA	*TERIS*	*Breast-feeding*
Beta-blockers			
Atenolol	D	U	caution
Metoprolol	C*	U	compatible
Nadolol	C*	U	compatible
Propranolol	C*	U	compatible
Timolol	C*	U	compatible
Adrenergic blockers			
Clonidine	C	U	compatible
Calcium channel blockers			
Diltiazem	C	U	compatible
Nifedipine	C	U	compatible
Nimodipine	C	U	uncertain
Verapamil	C	U	compatible

*Second or third trimester; FDA, Food and Drug Administration; TERIS, automated teratogen information resource

BREAST-FEEDING

Milk is a suspension of fat and protein in a carbohydrate–mineral solution. A nursing mother secretes 600 ml of milk per day that contains sufficient protein, fat and carbohydrate to meet the nutritional demands of the growing and developing infant[59]. The transport of a drug into breast milk depends on its lipid solubility, molecular weight, degree of ionization, protein binding and the presence or absence of active secretion[88]. Species differences in the composition of milk can result in differences in drug transfer. Since human milk (pH usually > 7.0) has a much higher pH than cow's milk (pH usually < 6.8), bovine drug transfer data may not be accurate in humans[59].

Many drugs can be detected in breast milk at levels that are not clinically significant to the infant. The concentration of drug in breast milk is a variable fraction of the maternal blood level. The infant dose is usually 1–2% of the maternal dose, which is usually trivial. However, any exposure to a toxic drug or potential allergen may be inappropriate[88].

Drug concentration in breast milk depends on drug characteristics (pK_a, lipid solubility, molecular weight, protein binding) and breast milk characteristics (composition and volume). Breast milk is given its unique physicochemical properties by the active transport of electro-

Table 20 Drugs and breast-feeding

(1)	Contraindicated
(2)	Require temporary cessation of breast-feeding
(3)	Effects unknown but may be of concern
(4)	Use with caution
(5)	Usually compatible

lytes, and the formation and excretion of lactose and proteins by glandular epithelial cells in the breast with passive diffusion of water. The volume produced depends on nutritional factors, the amount of milk removed by the suckling infant and the increase in mammary blood flow that occurs with breast-feeding. Volume production slowly increases from an average of 600 ml per day to 800 ml per day by the time the infant is 6 months old, and undergoes a diurnal variation, with the greatest quantity occurring in the morning. For the first 10 days of production, milk composition is characterized by a gradual increase in fat and lactose from a milk that is higher in protein content (colostrum).

Since most drugs are either weak acids or bases, the transfer across a biological membrane will be greatly influenced by the ionization characteristics (pK_a) and pH differences across the membrane. Because the pH of breast milk (7.0) is slightly lower than that of plasma (7.4), there is a tendency toward ion-trapping of basic compounds.

Classification of drugs used during lactation

The American Academy of Pediatrics Committee on Drugs has reviewed and categorized drugs for lactating women (Table 20)[79]. The following should be considered: is the drug necessary? If so, use the safest drug (e.g. acetaminophen instead of aspirin). If there is a possibility that a drug may present a risk to the infant (e.g. phenytoin, phenobarbital), consider measuring the blood level in the nursing infant. Drug exposure to the nursing infant may be minimized by having the mother take the medication just after completing a breast-feed.

The migraineur who is breast-feeding should avoid bromocriptine, ergotamine and lithium, and use sumatriptan, benzodiazepam, antidepressants and neuroleptics cautiously. Acetaminophen is compatible with breast-feeding and is preferred to aspirin. Moderate caffeine use is compatible with breast-feeding. However, accumulation may occur in infants whose mothers use excessive amounts. Narcotic use is compatible with breast-feeding. Phenobarbital has caused sedation in some nursing infants and it should be given to nursing mothers with caution.

SUMMARY

Migraine and TTH are primary headache disorders that commonly occur during pregnancy. Migraine sometimes occurs for the first time with pregnancy. The majority of migraineurs improve while pregnant; however, migraine often recurs postpartum. Some disorders that produce headache, such as stroke, cerebral venous thrombosis, eclampsia and SAH, occur more frequently during pregnancy. Diagnostic testing serves to exclude organic causes of headache, to confirm the diagnosis and to establish a baseline before treatment. If neurodiagnostic testing is indicated, the study that will provide the most information with the least fetal risk is the study of choice[8].

Drugs are commonly used during pregnancy despite insufficient knowledge about their effects on the growing fetus. Most drugs are not teratogenic. Adverse effects, such as spontaneous abortion, developmental defects and various postnatal effects, depend on the dose and route of administration and timing of the exposure relative to the period of fetal development.

While medication use should be limited, it is not absolutely contraindicated in pregnancy. In migraine, the risk of status migrainosus may be greater than the potential risk of the medication used to treat the pregnant patient. Non-pharmacologic treatment is the ideal solution; however, analgesics such as acetaminophen and narcotics can be used on a limited basis. Preventive therapy is a last resort.

References

1. Headache Classification Committee of the International Headache Society. Classification and diagnostic criteria for headache disorders, cranial neuralgia, and facial pain. *Cephalalgia* 1988;8:1–96
2. Silberstein SD, Young WB. Headache. In Pathy MSJ, ed. *Principles and Practice of Geriatric Medicine*. New York: John Wiley & Sons, 1998:733–46
3. Silberstein SD, Lipton RB, Dalessio DJ. Overview, diagnosis, and classification of headache. In Silberstein SD, Lipton RB, Dalessio DJ, eds. *Wolff's Headache and Other Head Pain*, 7th edn. New York: Oxford University Press, 2001:6–26
4. Silberstein SD, Saper JR, Freitag F. Migraine: diagnosis and treatment. In Silberstein SD, Lipton RB, Dalessio DJ, eds. *Wolff's Headache and Other Head Pain*, 7th edn. New York: Oxford University Press, 2001:121–237
5. Silberstein SD, Lipton RB, Goadsby PJ. *Headache in Clinical Practice*. Oxford: Isis Medical Media, 1998
6. Fox MV, Harms RW, Davis DH. Selected neurologic complications of pregnancy. *Mayo Clin Proc* 1990;65:1595–618
7. Hainline B. Headache. *Headache* 1994;12:443–60
8. Silberstein SD. Migraine and pregnancy. *Neurol Clin* 1997;15:209–31

9. Silberstein SD, Corbett JJ. The forgotten lumbar puncture. *Cephalalgia* 1993;13:212–13
10. Schwartz RB. Neurodiagnostic imaging of the pregnant patient. In *Neurologic Complications of Pregnancy*.
11. Stewart WF, Lipton RB, Celentano DD, Reed ML. Prevalence of migraine in the United States. Relation to age, income, race, and other sociodemographic factors. *J Am Med Assoc* 1992;267:64–9
12. Lipton RB, Silberstein SD, Stewart WF. An update on the epidemiology of migraine. *Headache* 1994;34:319–28
13. Silberstein SD. Headaches, pregnancy and lactation. In Yankowitz J, Niebyl JR, eds. *Drug Therapy in Pregnancy*, 3rd edn. Philadelphia: Lippincott Williams & Wilkins, 2001:231–46
14. Silberstein SD, Lipton RB. Overview of diagnosis and treatment of migraine. *Neurology* 1994;44:6–16
15. Silberstein SD, Young WB. Migraine aura and prodrome. *Semin Neurol* 1995;45:175–82
16. Silberstein SD. Migraine symptoms: results of a survey of self-reported migraineurs. *Headache* 1995;35:387–96
17. Selby G, Lance JW. Observation on 500 cases of migraine and allied vascular headaches. *J Neurol Neurosurg Psychiatry* 1960;23:23–32
18. Silberstein SD, Lipton RB. Chronic daily headache. In Goadsby PJ, Silberstein SD, eds. *Headache*. Newton: Butterworth-Heinemann, 1997: 201–25
19. Silberstein SD. Pharmacological management of cluster headache. *CNS Drugs* 1994;2:199–207
20. Labor DR, Mohr JP, Nichols FT, Tatemichi TK. Unilateral hyperhidrosis after cerebral infarction. *Neurology* 1988;38:1679–82
21. Forsyth PA, Posner JB. Headaches in patients with brain tumors. A study of 111 patients. *Neurology* 1993;43:1678–83
22. Britt RH. Brain abscess. In Wilkins RH, Rengachary SS, eds. *Neurosurgery*. New York: McGraw-Hill, 1985:1928–56
23. Ponder TM. Differential diagnosis of postdural puncture headache in the parturient. *Clin Forum Nurse Anesthetists* 1999;10:145–54
24. Vasdev GM, Chantigian RC. Pneumocephalus following the treatment of a postdural puncture headache with an epidural saline infusion. *J Clin Anesth* 1994;6:508–11
25. Abram SE, Cherwenka RW. Transient headache immediately following epidural steroid injection. *Anesthesiology* 1979;50:461–2
26. Kreitzer JM, Reed AP, Dauro AT, *et al*. Ascending back pain and headache during attempted epidural placement. *J Clin Anesth* 1991;3:414–17
27. Ravindran RS, Zandstra GC, Viegas OJ. Postpartum headache following regional analgesia: a symptom of cerebral venous thrombosis. *Can J Anaesth* 1989;36:705–7
28. Cohen JE, Godes J, Morales B. Postpartum bilateral subdural hematomas following spinal anesthesia: a case report. *Surg Neurol* 1997; 47:6–8
29. Eerola M, Kaukinen L, Kaukinen S. Fatal brain lesion following spinal anesthesia. *Acta Anesthesiol Scand* 1981;25:115–16

30. Jonsson LO, Einarsson P, Olsson GL. Subdural hematoma and spinal anesthesia. *Anesthesia* 1983;38:144–64
31. Pavlin DJ, McDonald JS, Child B, *et al*. Acute subdural hematoma: an unusual sequela to lumbar puncture. *Anesthesiology* 1979;51:338–40
32. Edelman JD, Wingard DW. Subdural hematomas after lumbar dural puncture. *Anesthesiology* 1980;52:166–7
33. Bader AM. Neurologic and neuromuscular disease. In Chestnut DH, ed. *Obstetric Anesthesia, Principles and Practice*. St Louis: Mosby Year Book, 1994:920–41
34. Chancellor MD, Wroe SJ. Migraine occurring for the first time in pregnancy. *Headache* 1990;30:224–7
35. Stein GS. Headaches in the first postpartum week and their relationship to migraine. *Headache* 1981;21:201–5
36. Somerville BW. A study of migraine in pregnancy. *Neurology* 1972;22: 824–8
37. Silberstein SD, Merriam GR. Sex hormones and headache. In Goadsby PJ, Silberstein SD, eds. *Headache*. Newton: Butterworth-Heinemann, 1997:143–73
38. Wright GD, Patel MK. Focal migraine and pregnancy. *Br Med J* 1986; 293:1557–8
39. Massey EW. Migraine during pregnancy. *Obstet Gynecol Surv* 1977;32: 693–6
40. Uknis A, Silberstein SD. Review article: migraine and pregnancy. *Headache* 1991;31:372–4
41. Lance JW, Anthony M. Some clinical aspects of migraine. *Arch Neurol* 1966;15:356–61
42. Callaghan N. The migraine syndrome in pregnancy. *Neurology* 1968;18: 197–201
43. Somerville BW. The role of estradiol withdrawal in the etiology of menstrual migraine. *Neurology* 1972;22:355–65
44. Ratinahirana H, Darbois Y, Bousser MG. Migraine and pregnancy: a prospective study in 703 women after delivery. *Neurology* 1990;40:437
45. Granella F, Sances G, Zanferrari C, Costa A, Martignoni E, Manzoni GC. Migraine without aura and reproductive life events: a clinical epidemiologic study in 1300 women. *Headache* 1993;33:385–9
46. Rasmussen BK. Migraine and tension-type headache in a general population: precipitating factors, female hormones, sleep pattern, and relation to lifestyle. *Pain* 1993;53:65–72
47. Chen TC, Leviton A. Headache recurrence in pregnant women with migraine. *Headache* 1994;34:107–10
48. Scharff L, Marcus DA, Turk DA. Headache during pregnancy and in the postpartum: a prospective study. *Headache* 1997;37:203–10
49. Maggioni F, Alessi C, Maggino T, Zanchin G. Headaches during pregnancy. *Cephalalgia* 1997;17:765–9
50. Granella F, Sances G, Pucci E, Nappi RE, Ghiotto N, Nappi G. Migraine with aura and reproductive life events: a case control study. *Cephalalgia* 2000;20:701–7
51. Sances G, Granella F, Nappi RE, *et al*. Course of migraine during pregnancy and postpartum: a prospective study. *Cephalalgia* 2003;23:197–205

52. Wainscott G, Volans GN. The outcome of pregnancy in women suffering from migraine. *Postgrad Med J* 1978;54:98–102
53. Olesen C, Steffensen FH, Sorensen HT, Nielsen GL, Olsen J. Pregnancy outcome following prescription for sumatriptan. *Headache* 1999;40:20–4
54. MacArthur C, Lewis M, Knox EG. Health after childbirth. *Br J Obstet Gynaecol* 1991;98:1193–204
55. Koren G, Pastuszak A, Ito S. Drugs in pregnancy. *N Engl J Med* 1998;338: 1128–37
56. Pitkin RM. Drug treatment of the pregnant woman: the state of the art. Presented at the *Food and Drug Administration Conference on Regulated Products and Pregnant Women*, Virginia, November 1995
57. Macklin R. Ethical conflicts and practical realities. Presented at the *Food and Drug Administration Conference on Regulated Products and Pregnant Women*, November 1994
58. Andrews EB. Use of observational methods to monitor the safety of marketed medications for risks of birth defects. Presented at the *Food and Drug Administration Conference on Regulated Products and Pregnant Women*, November 1994
59. Briggs GG, Freeman RK, Yaffe SJ. *Drugs in Pregnancy and Lactation*, 5th edn. Baltimore: Williams & Wilkins, 1994
60. Little BB, Gilstrap LC. Counseling and evaluation of the drug-exposed pregnant patient. In Gilstrap LC, ed. *Drugs and Pregnancy*. New York: Elsevier, 1992:23–9
61. Heinonen OP, Sloan S, Shapiro S. *Birth Defects and Drugs in Pregnancy*. Littleton: Publishing Sciences Group, 1977
62. Yankowitz J. Use of medications in pregnancy: general principles, teratology, and current developments. In Yankowitz J, Niebyl JR, eds. *Drug Therapy in Pregnancy*, 3rd edn. Philadelphia: Lippincott Williams & Wilkins, 2001:1–4
63. Medical Economics Company. *Physicians' Desk Reference*, 55th edn. Montvale, NJ: Thomson Healthcare, 2001
64. Friedman JM, Polifka JE. *Teratogenic Effects of Drugs: a Resource for Clinicians (TERIS)*. Baltimore: Johns Hopkins University Press, 1994
65. Friedman JM, Little BB, Brent RL, Cordero JF, Hanson JW, Shepard TH. Potential human teratogenicity of frequently prescribed drugs. *Obstet Gynecol* 1990;75:594–9
66. Daly LE, Kirke PN, Molloy A, Weir DG, Scott JM. Folate levels and neural tube defects: implications for prevention. *J Am Med Assoc* 1995;274: 1698–702
67. Ogawa Y, Kaneko S, Otani K, Fukushima Y. Serum folic acid levels in epileptic mothers and their relationship to congenital malformations. *Epilepsy Res* 1991;8:75–8
68. Jordan RL, Wilson JG, Shumacher HJ. Embryotoxicity of the folate antagonist methotrexate in rats and rabbits. *Teratology* 1977;15:73–80
69. Dansky LV, Andermann E, Rosenblatt D, Sherwin AL, Andermann F. Anticonvulsants, folate levels, and pregnancy outcome: a prospective study. *Ann Neurol* 1987;21:176–82
70. Reynolds EH. Anticonvulsants, folic acid and epilepsy. *Lancet* 1973;1: 1376–8

71. Wegner C, Nau H. Alteration of embryonic folate metabolism by valproic acid during organogenesis: implications for mechanism of teratogenesis. *Neurology* 1992;42:17–24
72. Metcalfe J, Stock MK, Barron DH. Maternal physiology during gestation. In Knobel E, Neill J, eds. *The Physiology of Reproduction*. New York: Raven Press, 1988:2145–74
73. Cunningham FG, MacDonald PC, Leveno KJ, Gant NF, Gilstrap LC. Maternal adaptations to pregnancy. In Cunningham FG, MacDonald PC, Leveno KJ, Gant NF, Gilstrap LC, eds. *Williams Obstetrics*, 19th edn. Connecticut: Appleton and Lange, 1993:209–46
74. Bailey RR, Rolleston GL. Kidney length and ureteric dilatation in the puerperium. *Br J Obstet Gynaecol* 1971;78:55
75. Chesley LC. Renal function during pregnancy. In Carey HM, ed. *Modern Trends in Human Reproductive Physiology*. London: Butterworth, 1963
76. Dunlop W. Serial changes in renal hemodynamics during normal human pregnancy. *Br J Obstet Gynaecol* 1981;88:1
77. Chaudhuri G. Pharmacokinetics in pregnancy. Presented at the *Food and Drug Administration Conference on Regulated Products and Pregnant Women*, November 1994
78. Yerby MS, Friel PN, McCormick K. Antiepileptic drug disposition during pregnancy. *Neurology* 1992;42:12–16
79. Murray L, Seger D. Drug therapy during pregnancy and lactation. *Emerg Med Clin North Am* 1994;12:129–49
80. Szeto HH. Kinetics of drug transfer to the fetus. *Clin Obstet Gynecol* 1993; 36:246–54
81. Raskin NH. Migraine treatment. In Raskin NH, ed. *Headache*, 2nd edn. New York: Churchill Livingstone, 1988
82. Silberstein SD. Appropriate use of abortive medication in headache treatment. *Pain Manage* 1991;4:22–8
83. Byron MA. Prescribing in pregnancy: treatment of rheumatic disease. *Br Med J* 1987;294:236–8
84. MacGregor A. Treatment of migraine during pregnancy. *IHS News Headache* 1994;4:3–9
85. Rayburn WF, Lavin JP. Drug prescribing for chronic medical disorders during pregnancy: an overview. *Am J Obstet Gynecol* 1986;155:565–9
86. Reiff-Eldridge R, Heffner CR, Ephross SA, Tennis PS, White AD, Andrews EB. Monitoring pregnancy outcomes after prenatal drug exposure through prospective pregnancy registries: a pharmaceutical company commitment. *Am J Obstet Gynecol* 2000;182:159–63
87. Källén B, Lygner PE. Delivery outcome in women who used drugs for migraine during pregnancy with special reference to sumatriptan. *Headache* 2001;41:351–6
88. Niebyl JR. Teratology and drugs in pregnancy and lactation. In Winters R, ed. *Danforth's Obstetrics and Gynecology*, 6th edn. New York: Lippincott, 1990

2

Cerebrovascular disease in pregnancy

S. Waddy and B. J. Stern

INTRODUCTION

Cerebrovascular disease in pregnancy and the postpartum period is an uncommon yet important cause of maternal and fetal morbidity, and causes between 3.5 and 26 instances of neurologic dysfunction per 100 000 deliveries[1,2]. During this period, complications from stroke include premature delivery[3], arterial and venous infarctions and hemorrhages. Importantly, more than 12% of maternal deaths have been attributed to stroke[4].

Pregnancy-associated stroke poses challenges to clinicians because of the difficulty in diagnosing the underlying cause, which includes known stroke-in-the-young factors as well as unique pregnancy-induced etiologies. Equally significant are adverse events caused by the potential fetal toxicity of diagnostic testing and the fetal toxicity of available treatments[3].

The patient's history and physical examination provide important information regarding the type of cerebrovascular event that may have occurred. As well, a thorough history and physical examination guide both diagnostic testing and acute treatment. Key historical points include the presence of pain, particularly headache or neck pain, and trauma. Furthermore, the presences of fluctuating neurologic symptoms, as well as the presence of seizures, confusion, a recent febrile illness and drug use, are also important to aid in determining the appropriate diagnosis and management. A complete past medical and family history should be obtained and include history of previous stroke or thrombosis, atherosclerosis risk factors, spontaneous abortions and possible collagen vascular diseases. The patient's medication and drug history may aid diagnosis as well, and should include a history of dietary supplementation.

On physical examination, attention to the funduscopic, cardiovascular and skin examinations as well as the neurologic examination are of vital significance. Funduscopic and eye evaluation may reveal evidence of disk edema from increased intracranial pressure, the presence of emboli or evidence of vasculitis. (A formal ophthalmologic evaluation may be needed.) The cardiovascular examination can demonstrate rhythm and rate disturbances, jugular venous distension and other signs of cardiac insufficiency or failure. The patient's skin should be examined for evidence of emboli, livido reticularis and decreased elasticity. A thorough neurologic evaluation is a necessity and should be performed not only to determine the localization and pathophysiology of the underlying problem, but also to determine the presence of clinical deterioration in the ensuing minutes, hours or days after a stroke.

Once the history has been obtained and the physical examination has been performed, diagnostic testing is usually required. For evaluation of stroke, several imaging studies are available to evaluate the parenchyma, vessels and extraparenchymal spaces. These include computerized tomography (CT) with or without ionic contrast, angiography (CTA) or venography (CTV), and magnetic resonance imaging (MRI) with or without contrast, angiography (MRA) or venography (MRV). Disease mechanism may also require evaluation by electrocardiography, transesophageal echocardiography, with or without agitated saline echo contrast, and transcranial Doppler sonography. In some cases, conventional arteriography may be needed to evaluate smaller-caliber vessels, degree of stenosis or presence of thrombus. A lumbar puncture may provide additional information regarding bleeding, infection and inflammation.

Each of the imaging studies discussed above has a potential role in the diagnosis of cerebrovascular disease and evaluation of the underlying etiology. Each also has limitations. The first limitation is length of time needed to perform the study, which may be important in the critically ill or unstable patient; CT/CTA/CTV requires minutes, compared to up to an hour for the multiple studies of MRI/MRA/MRV. Another difference between imaging studies is the ability to detect the suspected disease. Disease detection varies according to the location of disease as well as the length of time that the lesion has been present. CT provides limited visualization of the posterior fossa, particularly of infarction because of artifact; as well, detection of infarction may be limited during the hours after the event. Hemorrhage, on the other hand, is easily detected in most cases by head CT during the acute period. In contrast, MRI detection of infarction during the acute period is substantially better than CT, particularly when diffusion-weighted imaging is used; hemorrhage detection is improved as the patient progresses from the acute to subacute to chronic stage. It is important to note that not only the presence or absence of hemorrhage should be noted, but also the amount of edema, degree of mass effect and morphology of cisterns/ventricles should be evaluated for evidence of current or impending compromise.

Radiation exposure is always a concern to the clinician caring for the pregnant patient. CT has a risk of fetal radiation exposure, which can be minimized with appropriate abdominal shielding. This risk has not been shown to be present with magnetic imaging.

Even though imaging provides important information regarding stroke location, and at times etiology, other tests that should not be overlooked include hematologic studies and coagulation profiles.

CEREBRAL INFARCTION

Both arterial and venous infarctions are important causes of stroke, and account for the majority of cerebrovascular events in pregnancy and the postpartum period[5]. According to Jaigobin and Silver[5], 21 of 34 pregnant patients had strokes caused by either venous or arterial infarction; 13 of the 34 patients had hemorrhages of various causes. As found by Kittner and colleagues, infarction risk is not evenly distributed throughout pregnancy. This community-based, multihospital, retrospective study found that the relative risk of infarction increased from 0.7 during pregnancy to 8.7 during the postpartum period[6]. Etiologies for arterial infarction include vasculopathy, cardiogenic embolism and hematologic conditions. Venous infarctions may occur in patients who are dehydrated or have hyperviscosity syndromes, are infected or are hypercoagulable[5].

Vasculopathy

Vasculopathy is an important cause of arterial infarction in the general population and during pregnancy. Even though atherosclerosis is uncommon in young patients, it may cause stroke during pregnancy and should not be dismissed; however, the presence of atherosclerosis risk factors alone does not equate to a pathogenic role for atherosclerosis. In addition, if atherosclerosis is present, alternative causes may need to be evaluated. Other non-atherosclerotic vasculopathies include arterial dissection and fibromuscular dysplasia, moya moya disease and postpartum cerebral angiopathy.

Arterial dissection may be spontaneous or due to trauma. Not uncommonly, the underlying traumatic event may not be readily available in the patient's history, with the event occurring days to weeks prior to the neurologic event, or the trauma may seem insignificant to the patient, resulting in decreased reporting of the incident. As well, dissection may occur in patients with an underlying systemic vasculopathy, such as a collagen vascular disease. In most cases, an evaluation of the underlying etiology should be undertaken.

Moya moya disease is a progressive disorder that may be idiopathic or secondary to diseases that cause vascular injury such as sickle cell anemia. The hallmark of this disease is stenosis and eventual occlusion of the rostral carotid artery; many small, penetrating collateral vessels develop. Through several mechanisms, stroke, either infarction or particularly hemorrhage, may then occur.

Postpartum cerebral angiopathy is a rare and reversible disorder that results in the angiographic appearance of vessel narrowing[7]. Multiple vessels in the anterior and posterior circulations have been described as being involved. Even though the clinical phenotype of headache, seizure and focal neurologic deficits mimic eclampsia, which is described below, patients with postpartum cerebral angiopathy typically lack the findings of proteinuria and hypertension. The pathologic findings of Geraghty have shown that this appearance of lumen narrowing is explained by an endotheliopathy[8].

The long-term risk of re-infarction is decreased in patients with most forms of vasculopathy with antithrombotic therapy. The exceptions are arterial dissection and postpartum cerebral angiopathy. Management of acute arterial dissection includes anticoagulation and occasionally endovascular intervention[9]. Postpartum cerebral angiopathy is rare and information regarding appropriate treatment is limited; improvement has occurred with steroids and nimodipine, or other calcium antagonist therapy[7]. Treatment with hyperosmolar and hypervolemic therapy has also been used successfully[10].

Hematologic conditions

Several hematologic disorders result in stroke. These can involve alterations in the coagulation systems as well as erythrocytes and platelets.

A relative hypercoagulable state occurs in pregnancy, and during the first 3 weeks of the postpartum period[11].This hypercoagulable state is driven by an increase in thrombin formation beginning during the 12th week of pregnancy, and followed by alterations in the anticoagulation system in which antithrombin III (ATIII) and protein S decrease[12–14].

The endogenous anticoagulants are ATIII, protein C and protein S; while their roles in venous thrombosis in stroke in young patients have been established, their roles in arterial infarction are less clearly defined. Factor V Leiden mutation, which results in resistance to the activity of activated protein C and therefore skews the system toward coagulation, has also been established as a significant cause of venous thrombosis. The role of the factor V Leiden mutation in arterial infarction is even less clear than that of the anticoagulants ATIII, protein C and protein S. When testing of these anticoagulants is performed, care must be taken to check the activity of these anticoagulants rather than their levels. Either screening for activated protein C inhibition or direct mutation detection may test factor V Leiden.

Antiphospholipid antibodies (aPLs) are heterogeneous antibodies that lead to thrombosis. The aPLs, which include anticardiolipin (aCL) antibodies and lupus anticoagulants, may be responsible for venous or arterial thrombosis and should be suspected in patients who have experienced multiple fetal losses. Other characteristics that may be present include thrombocytopenia and cutaneous lesions such as livedo reticularis, cutaneous ulcerations and painful skin nodules[15]. A series of tests are required to confirm the presence of aPLs. aCL may be tested by enzyme-linked immunosorbent assay (ELISA) or radioimmunoassay. Detection of aCL immunoglobulin G (IgG) isotype in elevated amounts has been associated with thrombosis more so than IgM[16]. Lupus anticoagulant may be suspected in patients with a prolonged activated partial thromboplastin time. This should be confirmed through combination testing with either Russell viper venom or kaolin clotting times. If the patient tests positive for an aPL, it is important to determine whether the antibody is primary or secondary to an underlying disease, such as systemic lupus erythematosus.

Women with a known pre-pregnancy hypercoagulable state (such as ATIII, protein C or protein S deficiency or antiphospholipid syndrome, altered fibrinolysis or the factor V Leiden mutation) may have a greater risk of stroke during pregnancy because of the hypercoagulable state of pregnancy.

Altered coagulation should be explored in patients with a personal or family history of recurrent thromboses, recurrent spontaneous abortions or fetal losses not otherwise explained, and continued thrombosis despite adequate anticoagulation. In addition, the possibility of venous thrombosis from lower-extremity or pelvic vein thrombosis resulting in arterial emboli through a transcardiac mechanism should not be overlooked.

Other hematologic disorders that should be noted in pregnant patients include hemoglobinopathies and platelet disorders. These disorders are important etiologies, not only because of their causal relationship to stroke, as in the case of sickle cell crisis or thrombotic thrombocytopenic purpura, but also because of other secondary complications as in the case of fat embolus, which has been described in both hemoglobin SC and sickle cell disease or moya moya syndrome, as in the case of sickle cell disease[17,18].

The treatment of hematologic conditions varies depending on the underlying disease. Anticoagulation is typically indicated in hypercoagulable states. The hemoglobinopathies and platelet disorders require treatment directed at the underlying condition, which may, for example, include simple or exchange transfusion in the case of sickle cell anemia.

Cardiogenic

In Jaigobin and Silver's retrospective analysis[5], arterial stroke was caused by a cardiogenic source in more than one-third of the patients. The cardioembolic mechanisms of infarction may be divided into surface anomalies, conduction disturbances, inotropic failure and congenital cardiac defect. The surface anomalies and their causes are vast, and include bacterial and non-bacterial endocarditis, paradoxical embolism through a patent foramen ovale (PFO), mechanical valve and PFO with associated atrial septal aneurysm. The primary conduction disturbance of concern in stroke is atrial fibrillation. Even though inotropic failure may occur in the non-pregnant patient in the form of a pre-existing dilated cardiomyopathy, peripartum cardiomyopathy should be distinguished from the pre-existing form because of the possibility of inotropic improvement after delivery and improved survival rate at 5 years[19].

Peripartum cardiomyopathy is a rare cause of cerebral infarction. This cardiomyopathy occurs in women during their last month of pregnancy and during the first months postpartum, develops in women with no prior history of cardiac disease and leads to fulminate loss of left ventricular systolic function. This dysfunction may lead to thrombus formation and result in emboli. Anticoagulation is indicated for severe inotropic dysfunction. Additional medications and treatment such as salt reduction and vasodilating agents for afterload reduction in an effort to improve systolic function are generally required as well[20].

Other embolic sources and thrombosis causes

Reported instances of air embolus, fat embolus and amniotic fluid embolus have also occurred.

TREATMENT MODALITIES FOR ISCHEMIC STROKE

The goal of stroke treatment is to minimize neuronal loss or damage as well as prevent repeat occurrences of ischemia. Treatment of ischemic stroke during pregnancy requires consideration of many factors, including stroke etiology, maternal benefit, maternal risk and fetal toxicity. The primary treatments of ischemic stroke are anticoagulants and anti-thrombotics. Other treatments include thrombolytics and interventional procedures.

Anticoagulation

Anticoagulation prevents embolization, halts clot propagation and maintains luminal patency. Anticoagulation may be effective in both arterial and venous infarction. Indications for anticoagulation include atrial fibrillation, hypercoagulability, venous thrombosis, acute dissection and prophylaxis in patients with mechanical valves. Multiple routes of administration of anticoagulants are available including intravenous, subcutaneous and oral administration.

The available anticoagulants include unfractionated heparin (UH), heparin-like anticoagulants which include low-molecular-weight heparin (LMWH) and warfarin. These medications mediate clot inhibition by targeted inhibition of the various proteins of the coagulation cascade. Even though all of these agents have been shown to be effective in the treatment of ischemic stroke, they differ significantly in their adverse-effect profiles.

Heparin and heparin-like compounds: category C

Heparin and the heparin-like compounds have been shown to be effective in multiple stroke subtypes. A major benefit of UH and heparin-like compounds is their rapid onset of action. Intravenous administration has an immediate effect, while subcutaneous administration causes a delay of a few hours. Another benefit to pregnant patients is decreased teratogenicity because of lack of transplacental crossing. Even though heparin and the heparin-like compounds are similar, their differences in modes of action and adverse reactions should be highlighted.

Heparin and its derivative LMWH are heterogeneous glycosaminoglycans which bind to ATIII, a protein in the anticoagulation system, to inhibit coagulation selectively[21,22]. Binding of these medications to ATIII causes a conformational change that enhances ATIII's ability to inactivate various coagulation proteins. UH and LMWH bind to ATIII and form a complex with proteins in the coagulation cascade. In the case of UH, the complex is formed with activated thrombin and to a lesser extent factors Xa and IXa; in contrast, LMWH forms the complex with factor Xa. Inactivation of these compounds leads to inhibition of coagulation and hence anticoagulation.

UH and LMWH differ not only in the targeted protein for anticoagulation but also in their adverse-effects profile, laboratory monitoring and route of administration. Two forms of heparin-induced thrombocytopenia occur. The early, reversible benign form is not discussed here. The IgG-mediated heparin-induced thrombocytopenia (HIT) may be life-threatening, and is associated with thrombotic complications despite anticoagulation. In this syndrome, which begins 5–15 days after heparin administration in the heparin-naive patient, a rapid thrombocytopenia occurs, reducing platelet counts and increasing the risk of thrombosis through platelet activation. HIT is estimated to occur in approximately 1% of patients receiving UH. HIT occurs less often in patients treated with LMWH; however, once HIT occurs in a patient, LMWH cannot be used. Because of the possibility of HIT occurring with either medication, periodic platelet monitoring during administration is required.

Another adverse event that occurs with administration of UH or LMWH is osteoporosis. Heparin-associated osteoporosis ranges from subclinical reduction of bone density to clinically evident fractures. This disorder arises less frequently in the patient receiving LMWH, compared with UH, and occurs in a time-dependent fashion. The mechanism of osteoporosis development is not entirely understood.

In terms of efficacy, both UH and LMWH are efficacious in the treatment of embolic disease in patients with infarction. Because of the difference in mechanisms of action of UH and LMWH, these medications require different monitoring methods. The activated partial thromboplastin time (aPTT) is based on the final pathway of thrombin. Because of UH's inactivation of factor IIa, the aPTT can be used for its monitoring. The aPTT is not appropriate for monitoring LMWH because inhibition of the coagulation cascade with LMWH is through factor Xa rather than IIa. Monitoring of LMWH requires measurement of trough levels of anti-Xa activity or heparin levels. During pregnancy, monitoring and dose adjustments may be difficult because of the continuous changes in maternal volume of distribution. Therefore, frequent monitoring throughout pregnancy is required.

Appropriate dosing of UH and LMWH depends on utilizing symptomatic or at-risk protocols. For prophylactic (at-risk) therapy, UH at 7500–10 000 IU should be given every 12 h, with an aPTT goal of 1.5 times the control, and should be evaluated at 6 h post-injection. If plasma heparin levels are measured, the target level is 0.2–0.4 IU/ml. The therapeutic treatment dose for LMWH varies, depending on the preparation used. Enoxaparin, for example, should be titrated to a goal anti-Xa activity of 0.1 to 0.2 U/ml for at-risk treatment, and a more aggressive goal of 0.6–0.8 U/ml for symptomatic treatment, with trough levels of greater than 0.2 U/ml[23].

Warfarin: category X

Vitamin K is a cofactor needed for the post-translational modification of several coagulation and anticoagulation factors. These factors include prothrombin, factor VII, factor IX and factor X as well as several factors in the regulatory pathway, which include protein C and protein S. The oral anticoagulant warfarin mechanistically inhibits the ability of post-translational carboxylation to occur, which results in anticoagulation. Anticoagulation with warfarin has been shown to be effective in several etiologies of venous and arterial disease. Limitations in its use in pregnant patients exist because of warfarin's adverse reaction profile. Unlike heparin, warfarin may result in complications owing to transplacental crossing of medication. These complications predominate during organogenesis (weeks 6–12 of gestation). Other complications include maternal bleeding as well as fetal bleeding, spontaneous abortions and stillbirths.

If warfarin is selected as a treatment, then dosing with an International Normalized Ratio (INR) goal of 2.0–3.0 is typically appropriate; however, in high-risk patients such as individuals with mechanical prosthetic valves, some studies advocate higher levels (2.5–4.0).

Antithrombotics

While anticoagulants target the coagulation system, antithrombotics inhibit the ability of platelets to initiate clot formation and aggregation.

Aspirin: category D

Aspirin's antithrombotic activity occurs through cyclo-oxygenase inhibition, resulting in decreased production of thromboxane-A_2 on the platelet surface, causing platelet aggregation inhibition. Aspirin has been found to be an effective therapy for stroke treatment in the non-pregnant patient; however, it has been shown to have restricted use in the pregnant patient because of the development of other effective antithrombotic medications with fewer adverse events. These adverse effects include peripartum bleeding, prolonged pregnancy and labor, and stillbirths and fetal intracranial hemorrhage. These events appear to be dose-dependent, with low-dose aspirin (60 mg) being found to be relatively safe. Abruptio placentae may occur at an increased rate at any dose[24].

Clopidogrel: category B

Clopidogrel is an effective antithrombotic agent frequently used in non-pregnant patients for stroke prophylaxis. Clopidogrel inhibits platelet aggregation through indirect adenosine diphosphate/glycoprotein complex inhibition. It has not been found to cause significant fetotoxicity in animals at extremely high doses; however, adequate studies in human pregnancies have not occurred.

Dipyridamole and aspirin: category B (dipyridamole) and category D (aspirin)

Aspirin and extended-release dipyridamole is yet another effective antithrombotic medication used in the treatment of stroke[25]. Dipyridamole's action alters the local environment of platelets and the endothelium of vessels through adenosine uptake blockage in platelets. This drives the formation of cyclic adenosine monophosphate, and inhibits the platelet's aggregation response to other factors such as collagen and adenosine diphosphate. Low-dose aspirin, which inhibits cyclo-oxygenase inhibition of platelets, has an additive effect to that of extended-release dipyridamole.

Studies regarding the safety of dipyridamole are limited; however, dipyridamole has not been found to cause significant teratogenic effects in animals at moderate doses. Owing to its combination with aspirin, this medication may have limited use in the pregnant patient, particularly during the third trimester.

Acute infarction

During the last decade, the rapid administration of tissue plasminogen activator (tPA) has been responsible for decreasing the morbidity and mortality of ischemic stroke in patients who meet criteria for treatment. Pregnant patients were excluded from the major tPA trial for stroke[26]. Pregnant patients have been given tPA for non-stroke thromboembolic events. tPA has also been administered in pregnant patients with significant neurologic dysfunction. Alternatives include intra-arterial thrombolysis and mechanical clot disruption. Intra-arterial urokinase for basilar artery thrombosis[27] and intra-arterial recombinant tPA to the middle cerebral artery have been given successfully in individual cases[28]. These procedures are under current investigation primarily in non-pregnant patients; however, limited coagulation manipulation with direct treatment of the active thromboembolic process make these interventions intriguing treatment alternatives.

Thrombolytics

Tissue plasminogen activator: category C

Plasmin destroys fibrin strands. tPA accelerates the production of plasmin through enhanced plasminogen conversion to plasmin. Determination of the effects of tPA on pregnancy have not been adequately evaluated in humans or animals.

Intracranial venous thrombosis

Venous thrombosis causes ischemic and hemorrhagic strokes. Even though it is an uncommon disorder in young patients, its significance increases during pregnancy. In a multistate data analysis from the Healthcare Cost and Utilization Project, the risk of intracranial venous thrombosis was found to be 11.66 cases per 100 000 deliveries[29].

The hallmarks of the disorder are headache due to increased intracranial pressure or focal hemorrhage, seizures and focal neurologic impairment. Lanska and Kryscio's evaluation[29] revealed that patients with hypertension, dehydration and infections other than pneumonia and influenza were significantly more likely to have intracerebral venous thrombosis. Correct diagnosis of intracerebral venous thrombosis is difficult without the appropriate imaging studies (CTV or MRV). With close inspection, the thrombosed vein may be present on CT or MRI with and without contrast enhancement. Rapid evaluation and treatment are necessary to prevent neurologic deterioration. This deterioration may occur through progressive infarction or hemorrhage, persisting seizures and rising intracranial pressure. Effective treatment requires inhibition of thrombus propagation as well as seizure control and lowering of increased intracranial pressure. In the non-critical patient, thrombus propagation can be managed with anticoagulation[30]. If deterioration occurs, invasive procedures may be considered. Both mechanical disruption of the clot and selective intrasinus thrombolysis have been used in limited series of non-pregnant patients[31].

Eclampsia

The hallmark of eclampsia is pregnancy-induced hypertension with proteinuria, and generalized tonic–clonic convulsions developing during the peripartum period. Typically, eclampsia occurs in the 24 h before or after delivery[32]. On rare occasions, women may develop eclampsia during the month following delivery[33,34]. Neurologic symptoms occur because of seizures, ischemic infarction, hemorrhage or posterior leukoencephalopathy. Treatment of eclampsia includes blood pressure and seizure control with magnesium sulfate. In the event of stroke, the eclampsia should be treated and fetal delivery expedited, if possible. Monitoring and treatment of increased intracranial pressure may be necessary[35].

Hemorrhage

Even though hemorrhage occurs slightly less often than arterial and venous infarction, it is associated with worse morbidity and mortality rates in the pregnant patient. In the 20-year retrospective analysis by Witlin and colleagues, 20 patients were found to have postpartum stroke. All deaths that occurred due to stroke were caused by intracerebral hemorrhage[36].

A variety of disorders cause hemorrhage during pregnancy and the postpartum period; these include the above-discussed disorders of moya moya disease, eclampsia and venous thrombosis. Other disorders that result in hemorrhage include aneurysmal subarachnoid hemorrhage (SAH), arteriovenous malformations (AVMs) and pituitary apoplexy. A combination of supportive therapy including blood pressure and intracranial pressure monitoring, medications and invasive procedures may be needed in the management of these patients.

Aneurysmal subarachnoid hemorrhage

The presenting complaint of pregnant patients with aneurysmal SAH is 'the worst headache of my life'. The patient's condition may vary from normal to comatose. Determination of the presence of an aneurysmal SAH may require not only neurologic imaging but also lumbar puncture. Aneurysm rupture may occur at any time during pregnancy, but occurs most frequently during the third trimester to the early postpartum period.

The definitive treatment of aneurysmal SAH is protection of the aneurysm by either surgical clipping or coiling. Aggressive treatment is required because of the significant re-rupture rate, as well as high maternal morbidity and mortality with non-treatment; improved maternal and fetal outcomes have occurred with early protection of the aneurysm. Other treatment goals of patients with aneurysmal rupture include decreasing the risk of vasospasm, monitoring and treating hydrocephalus, and prevention of seizures, when needed.

Vasospasm is an important cause of morbidity and mortality in patients with SAH. When it occurs, one-third will become symptomatic; of those, nearly one-third will die and one-third will have permanent disability without corrective treatment[37]. Vasospasm detection may require frequent monitoring with transcranial Doppler sonography, or imaging of the intracranial vessels. Hypervolemia, hemodilution and hypertensive (HHH) therapy may be required to treat vasospasm, but must be used with caution in pregnancy because they expand the blood volume. In the non-pregnant patient, HHH therapy reduced the incidence of ischemic deficits by nearly half[38].

The calcium channel antagonist nimodipine has also been shown to improve patient outcomes. Nimodipine is a category C medication; however, aneurysmal SAH is infrequent during organogensis, occurring more commonly during the third trimester and postpartum period. If vasospasm should occur then angioplasty should be considered.

There is limited evidence regarding modes of delivery in the patient with an aneurysm. Cesarean section should be considered in a patient with a symptomatic unruptured and untreated aneurysm. If the aneurysm is asymptomatic and unruptured or treated with coiling or clipping, then either vaginal delivery or Cesarean section may be an option. A symptomatic ruptured and untreated aneurysm in a patient rapidly approaching delivery is the most worrying situation, and warrants consideration of Cesarean section.

Cerebral arteriovenous malformation

While aneurysms more commonly cause SAH, cerebral AVMs typically result in intraparenchymal hemorrhage and occasionally cause SAH. Pathologically, AVMs are congenital masses of abnormal arteries and veins that lack an intervening capillary bed. These masses consist of friable vessels that may bleed. Bleeding or hemorrhage may lead to seizures, headaches or focal neurologic deficits.

Even though untreated AVMs may hemorrhage at any time during one's life with a 2–4 % annual hemorrhage rate, they have been found to have an increased rate of hemorrhage during pregnancy, particularly during the second trimester, partum and postpartum periods.

An AVM that has previously hemorrhaged and has not undergone treatment has a significant risk of re-hemorrhage[39]. Guidelines for when treatment should be given are not well defined; however, treatment options during pregnancy include either resection or embolization. (Stereotactic radiosurgery provides no significant protection during this period because of the interval of latent effect, which is approximately 2 years.) The optimal mode of delivery has not been well established, and should be based on obstetric considerations.

Pituitary apoplexy

A rare but important form of hemorrhage occurs in pituitary apoplexy. Symptoms include the sudden onset of severe headache (which is most commonly retro-orbital), visual disturbance with ophthalmoplegia and potential progression to altered consciousness. Pathologically, when hemorrhage into the pituitary gland occurs, a pre-existing pituitary adenoma may be identified.

This syndrome is of importance because of the clinical similarities to other causes of hemorrhage, such as aneurysmal SAH. As well, the complications and treatment of this disorder are distinct from other causes of hemorrhage. The initial management of pituitary apoplexy includes close monitoring of the progression of neurologic deficits and alteration in consciousness; this requires frequent evaluation of the patient's visual fields for red desaturation defects or defects found with formal visual field testing. Evaluation of the pituitary hormones is important as well as monitoring for hyponatremia, which may lead to alteration in consciousness.

Conservative management with monitoring and treatment of electrolyte imbalance and administration of glucocorticoids may be needed. Surgical intervention with transphenoidal decompression of the sella is used when neuro-ophthalmological indications occur[40].

References

1. Wiebers DO, Whisnant JP. The incidence of stroke among pregnant women in Rochester, Minn, 1955 through 1979. *J Am Med Assoc* 1985; 254:3055–7
2. Rochat RW, Koonin LM, Atrash HK, Jewett JF. Maternal mortality in the United States: report from the Maternal Mortality Collaborative. *Obstet Gynecol* 1988;72:91–7
3. Sharshar T, Lamy C, Mas JL. Incidence and causes of strokes associated with pregnancy and puerperium. A study in public hospitals of Ile de France. Stroke in Pregnancy Study Group. *Stroke* 1995;26:930–6
4. Simolke GA, Cox SM, Cunningham FG. Cerebrovascular accidents complicating pregnancy and the puerperium. *Obstet Gynecol* 1991;78:37–42
5. Jaigobin C, Silver FL. Stroke and pregnancy. *Stroke* 2000;31:2948–51
6. Kittner SJ, Stern BJ, Feeser BR, *et al.* Pregnancy and the risk of stroke. *N Engl J Med* 1996;335:768–74
7. Lee KY, Sohn YH, Kim SH, *et al.* Basilar artery vasospasm in postpartum cerebral angiopathy. *Neurology* 2000;54:2003–5
8. Geraghty JJ. Fatal puerperal cerebral vasospasm and stroke in a young woman. *Neurology* 1991;41:1145–7
9. Malek AM, Higashida RT, Phatouros CC, *et al.* Endovascular management of extracranial carotid artery dissection achieved using stent angioplasty. *AJNR Am J Neuroradiol* 2000;21:1280–92
10. Akins PT. Postpartum cerebral vasospasm treated with hypervolemic therapy. *Am J Obstet Gynecol* 1996;175:1386–8
11. Dahlman T, Hellgren M, Blomback M. Changes in blood coagulation and fibrinolysis in the normal puerperium. *Gynecol Obstet Invest* 1985;20: 37–44
12. Pinto S, Abbate R, Rostago C, *et al.* Increased thrombin generation in normal pregnancy. *Acta Eur Fertil* 1988;19:263–7
13. Malm J, Laurell M, Dahlback B. Changes in the plasma levels of vitamin K-dependent proteins C and S and of C4b-binding protein during pregnancy and oral contraception. *Br J Haematol* 1988;68:437–41
14. de Boer K, ten Cate JW, Sturk A, *et al.* Enhanced thrombin generation in normal and hypertensive pregnancy. *Am J Obstet Gynecol* 1989;160: 95–100

15. Gibson GE, Su WP, Pittelkow MR. Antiphospholipid syndrome and the skin. *J Am Acad Dermatol* 1997;36:970–82
16. Tanne D. Anticardiolipin antibodies and their associations with cerebrovascular risk factors. *Neurology* 1999;52:1368–73
17. Horton DP, Ferriero DM, Mentzer WC. Nontraumatic fat embolism syndrome in sickle cell anemia. *Pediatr Neurol* 1995;12:77–80
18. Rinkel GJ, Wijdicks EF, Hene RJ. Stroke in relapsing thrombotic thrombocytopenic purpura. *Stroke* 1991;22:1087–9
19. Felker GM, Thompson RE, Hare JM, *et al.* Underlying causes and long-term survival in patients with initially unexplained cardiomyopathy. *N Engl J Med* 2000;342:1077–84
20. Reimold S, Rutherford J. Peripartum cardiomyopathy. *N Engl J Med* 2001;344:1629–30
21. Beguin S, Lindhout T, Hemker HC. The mode of action of heparin in plasma. *Thromb Haemost* 1988;60:457–62
22. Bjork I, Lindahl U. Mechanism of the anticoagulant action of heparin. *Mol Cell Biochem* 1982;48:161–82
23. Boneu B. Low molecular weight heparin therapy: is monitoring needed? *Thromb Haemost* 1994;72:330
24. Sibai BM, Caritis SN, Thom E, *et al.* Prevention of preeclampsia with low-dose aspirin in healthy, nulliparous pregnant women. The National Institute of Child Health and Human Development Network of Maternal–Fetal Medicine Units. *N Engl J Med* 1993;329:1213–18
25. Forbes CD. Secondary stroke prevention with low-dose aspirin, sustained release dipyridamole alone and in combination. ESPS Investigators. European Stroke Prevention Study. *Thromb Res* 1998;92:S1–6
26. The National Institute of Neurological Disorders and Stroke rt-PA Stroke Study Group. Tissue plasminogen activator for acute ischemic stroke. *N Engl J Med* 1995;333:1581–7
27. Cincotta RB, Davis SM, Gerraty RP, *et al.* Thrombolytic therapy for basilar artery thrombosis in the puerperium. *Am J Obstet Gynecol* 1995;173: 967–9
28. Elford K, Leader A, Wee R, *et al.* Stroke in ovarian hyperstimulation syndrome in early pregnancy treated with intra-arterial rt-PA. *Neurology* 2002;59:1270–2
29. Lanska DJ, Kryscio RJ. Risk factors for peripartum and postpartum stroke and intracranial venous thrombosis. *Stroke* 2000;31:1274–82
30. Stam J, de Bruijn S, deVeber G. Anticoagulation for cerebral sinus thrombosis. *Stroke* 2003;34:1054–5
31. Smith AG, Cornblath WT, Deveikis JP. Local thrombolytic therapy in deep cerebral venous thrombosis. *Neurology* 1997;48:1613–19
32. Lubarsky SL, Barton JR, Friedman SA, *et al.* Late postpartum eclampsia revisited. *Obstet Gynecol* 1994;83:502
33. Brown CEL, Cunningham FG, Pritchard JA. Convulsions in hypertensive, proteinuric primiparas more than 24 hours after delivery: eclampsia or some other cause. *J Reprod Med* 1987;32:499
34. Lubarsky SL, Barton JR, Friedman SA, *et al.* Late postpartum eclampsia revisited. *Obstet Gynecol* 1994;83:502

35. Cunningham FG. Blindness associated with preeclampsia and eclampsia. *Am J Obstet Gynecol* 1995;172:1291–8
36. Witlin A, Mattar F, Sibai B. Postpartum stroke: a twenty-year experience. *Am J Obstet Gynecol* 2000;183:83–8
37. Dorsch NW. Therapeutic approaches to vasospasm in subarachnoid hemorrhage. *Curr Opin Crit Care* 2002;8:128–33
38. Dorsch NWC. A review of cerebral vasospasm in aneurysmal subarachnoid hemorrhage. II: Management. *J Clin Neurosci* 1994;1:78–92
39. Pollock B. Factors that predict the bleeding risk of cerebral arteriovenous malformations. *Stroke* 1996;27:1–6
40. Randeva H. Classical pituitary apoplexy; clinical features, management and outcome. *Clin Endocrinol* 1999;51:181–8

3

Pregnancy in women with epilepsy

P. B. Pennell

INTRODUCTION

Epilepsy is the most common major neurologic disorder in pregnancy requiring continuous treatment. Recent indications are that antiepileptic drug (AED) use occurs in 0.4–0.6% of all pregnancies[1,2], but this figure may increase as we see the emergence of AED use for other illnesses including headache, mood disorders and chronic pain. Most of the principles outlined below about AED use during pregnancy can be extrapolated to women with any disorder treated with these agents.

Although the vast majority of women with epilepsy have a normal pregnancy with favorable outcomes, they have increased maternal and fetal risks compared with the general population. Careful planning and management of any pregnancy in a woman with epilepsy is essential to minimize these risks. The reduction of these risks begins with preconceptional planning. The initial visit between the physician and a woman with epilepsy of child-bearing age should include a discussion about family planning. Topics should include effective birth control, the importance of planned pregnancies with AED optimization and folate supplementation prior to conception, obstetric complications and teratogenicity of AEDs versus the risks of seizures during pregnancy. The goal is effective control of maternal seizures with the least risk to the fetus.

BIRTH CONTROL FOR WOMEN ON ANTIEPILEPTIC DRUGS

Careful planning requires effective birth control. Many of the AEDs induce the hepatic cytochrome P450 system, which is also the primary metabolic pathway of the sex steroid hormones. The resulting increased

Table 1 Antiepileptic drug effects on hormonal contraceptive agents

Lowers hormone levels	*No significant effects*
Phenobarbital	ethosuximide
Phenytoin	valproate
Carbamazepine	gabapentin
Primidone	lamotrigine
Topiramate	tiagabine
Oxcarbazepine	levetiracetam
	zonisamide

enzymatic activity can lead to rapid clearance of steroid hormones and allow ovulation in women taking oral contraceptives or other hormonal forms of birth control[3,4]. An estradiol dose of 50 μg or its equivalent for 21 days of each cycle should be prescribed when using oral contraceptive agents with the enzyme-inducing AEDs[5]. Patients need to be warned that mid-cycle bleeding indicates possible birth-control failure, but its absence does not indicate adequate birth-control efficacy. Table 1 lists the effects of individual AEDs on hormonal contraceptive agents[4,6,7]. Subdermal levonorgestrel (Norplant®) also has a higher failure rate with these AEDs[8]. Intramuscular medroxyprogesterone provides higher dosages of progestin but still may require dosing at 8–10-week intervals rather than 12-week intervals. This has not yet been fully evaluated for women on AEDs.

FETAL ANTICONVULSANT SYNDROME

Offspring of women with epilepsy are at increased risk for intrauterine growth restriction, minor anomalies, major congenital malformations, cognitive dysfunction, microcephaly and infant mortality[9–12]. The term 'fetal anticonvulsant syndrome' is used to include various combinations of these findings, and has been described with virtually all of the AEDs[13].

Intrauterine growth restriction results in low birth weight (< 2500 g) in 7–10% of infants born to women with epilepsy[9,10], and is even more prevalent in infants exposed to polytherapy[14].

Minor anomalies

Minor anomalies are defined as structural deviations from the norm that do not constitute a threat to health. Minor anomalies affect 6–20% of infants born to women with epilepsy, an approximately two-fold increased rate compared with the general population[15]. Minor anomalies seen in infants of mothers on AEDs include distal digital and nail hypoplasia and the midline craniofacial anomalies, including ocular hypertelorism, broad nasal bridge, short upturned nose, altered lips, epicanthal folds and low hairline[15,16]. Many of the craniofacial anomalies are outgrown by age 5 years.

Major malformations

Major malformations are defined as an abnormality of an essential anatomical structure present at birth that interferes significantly with function and/or requires major intervention. Major malformations occur in 2–3% of general population births; reported rates in offspring of women with epilepsy range from 1.25 to 11.5%, with the combined estimates yielding a rate of 4–6%[5,11,15,17,18].

Major malformations (Table 2) most commonly associated with AED exposure include congenital heart disease, cleft lip/palate, neural tube defects and urogenital defects[15,16]. The congenital heart defects include atrial septal defect, ventricular septal defect, tetralogy of Fallot, coarctation of the aorta, patent ductus arteriosus and pulmonary stenosis. The neural tube defects usually consist of spina bifida and not anencephaly, but tend to be severe open defects frequently complicated by hydrocephaly and other midline defects[19]. Urogenital defects commonly involve glandular hypospadias.

Risks with AED polytherapy during pregnancy

Studies of pregnancy in women with epilepsy consistently demonstrate an increased risk for malformations with use of AED polytherapy[20–27]. The rate of major malformations has been reported to be as high as 25% in infants of women taking four or more AEDs[22]. One study in Japan analyzed 172 deliveries. The 31 infants exposed to AED monotherapy had a malformation rate of 6.5%, whereas the 141 infants exposed to

Table 2 Major malformations in infants of women with epilepsy

	General population (%)	*Infants of women with epilepsy (%)*
Congenital heart defects	0.5	1.5–2
Cleft lip/palate	0.15	1.4
Neural tube defects	0.1	1–3.8 (VPA) 0.5–1 (CBZ)
Urogenital defects	0.7	1.7

VPA, valproic acid; CBZ, carbamazepine

polytherapy had a malformation rate of 15.6% ($p = 0.01$)[25]. Comparison of two cohorts of patients from different intervals at the same Canadian institution found that the prevalence of major malformations was significantly different between groups (24.1% vs. 8.8%; $p < 0.01$), and the decreased prevalence correlated with the proportion of patients receiving AED monotherapy and a smaller mean number of drugs[24]. In a prospective study of the effects of AEDs in pregnant women with epilepsy in south-east France, the rate of malformations was higher in infants exposed to polytherapy (15%) than in those exposed to monotherapy (5%) ($p < 0.01$)[27]. These consistent results have led to current guidelines recommending monotherapy during pregnancy[5,15].

Risks with AED monotherapies during pregnancy

Findings of the fetal anticonvulsant syndrome have been described in association with virtually all of the AEDs, but there are subtle differences in the likelihood of specific malformations with the different AEDs. Lindhout and colleagues[22] described a difference in the types of major malformations seen with changes in prescribing practices in a comparison between two cohorts. The older cohort (1972–79) included more women taking phenobarbital, primidone and phenytoin than the later cohort; the features seen in this older cohort were congenital heart defects, facial clefts, developmental retardation and minor anomalies. In the newer cohort (1981–85), the prescribing of phenobarbital, primidone and phenytoin had decreased, and monotherapy with valproic acid or carbamazepine had increased. The congenital anomalies identified in the newer cohort most frequently were spinal defects and glandular hypospadias.

The relative risks for neural tube defects with carbamazepine and valproate are approximately 10 and 20 times those of the general population, respectively[28,29]. One analysis pooling data from five prospective studies suggested that the absolute risk with valproate monotherapy may be as high as 3.8% for neural tube defects, and that offspring of women receiving >1000 mg/day of valproate were especially at increased risk[20]. More recent collaborative studies have supported the significant dose–response relationship for valproate, with higher risks associated with doses above 1000 mg/day or with levels above 70 μg/ml[18,26,30].

With the exception of neural tube defects, no clear differences in other teratogenic risks for any of the AEDs have been demonstrated[13,31]. The American Academy of Neurology practice parameter summary statement in 1998 recommended that 'the AED most appropriate for seizure type and the drug producing optimal control with least side-effects remains the AED of choice for women with epilepsy'[5].

If a woman is at high risk for bearing a child with a neural tube defect because of her personal or family history, then valproic acid and carbamazepine should be chosen only if other AEDs are ineffective.

Currently ongoing prospective pregnancy registries hope to provide better information about the relative risks of each AED. Recent prospective data from the North American AED Pregnancy Registry are available for phenobarbital and valproic acid[32–34]. Of the 79 women receiving phenobarbital monotherapy, five of the infants had confirmed major malformations (6.3%; 95% confidence interval (CI) 2.1–14.2%), while only 1.62% of pregnancies with no AED exposure had malformations[34]. In first-trimester valproic acid monotherapy exposures (n = 123), major birth defects occurred in 8.8% of infants, compared with 2.8% in infants exposed to other AED monotherapies and 1.6% in external control infants (relative risk 5.43, 95% CI 3.09–9.55)[33].

The most recent results from the lamotrigine pregnancy registry[35] are based on 200 monotherapy exposures during the first trimester resulting in a live birth. Four of the newborns had a detected major malformation, resulting in a major malformation rate of 2.0% (95% CI 0.6–5.4%). Although this is still an insufficient sample size for reaching definitive conclusions about the possible teratogenic risk of lamotrigine, the results are encouraging for lamotrigine monotherapy. Notably, the combination of lamotrigine and valproic acid carried an especially high risk, with a major malformation rate of 12.1% (95% CI 5.4–23.9%).

The teratogenic effects of most of the other new AEDs are unknown at this time. Human birth defects have also been reported with oxcarbazepine, topiramate, gabapentin, tiagabine, levetiracetam and zonisamide, but accurate denominators are not available to calculate rates.

Prenatal screening

Prenatal screening should be offered to all women with epilepsy to detect any fetal major malformations. Neural tube defects should be screened in combination with maternal serum α-fetoprotein at 15–22 weeks and expert, targeted level II (structural) ultrasound at 16–20 weeks[5]. When performed together, these tests can identify over 95% of fetuses with open neural tube defects[36,37]. Amniocentesis (with measurements of amniotic fluid α-fetoprotein and acetylcholinesterase) should be offered if these tests are equivocal, increasing the sensitivity for detection of neural tube defects to greater than 99%. Detailed sonographic imaging of the fetal heart can be performed at 18–20 weeks' gestation and may be followed by fetal echocardiography if visualization is suboptimal. This approach can detect up to 85% of prenatally diagnosable cardiac abnormalities[37]. Careful imaging of the fetal face for cleft lip and palate can also be performed at 18–20 weeks' gestational age, although the accuracy of prenatal diagnosis is less established[37]. If the patient's weight gain and fundal growth do not appear appropriate, serial sonography should be performed to assess fetal size and amniotic fluid[38].

Neurodevelopmental outcome

The majority of studies investigating cognitive outcome in children of women with epilepsy report an increased risk of mental deficiency, affecting 1.4–6% of children of women with epilepsy, compared with 1% of controls[9,39]. Several studies have demonstrated increased risk for poor cognitive outcome with *in utero* exposure to AED polytherapy in particular[21,40–42]. Exposure during the last trimester may actually be the most detrimental[43], and verbal scores on neuropsychometric measures may be selectively more involved[11,40,44].

Associations between cognitive impairment and a variety of other factors have also been reported, including seizures[45], a high number of minor anomalies, major malformations, decreased maternal education, impaired mother–child relationships and maternal partial seizure disorder[46].

A recent retrospective survey suggested an especially high risk associated with valproic acid for the neurodevelopment of children exposed *in utero*[41]. Compared with children of women with epilepsy on no AEDs, the odds ratios for additional educational needs were 1.49 for all children exposed to AEDs *in utero* and 3.4 for children exposed to valproic acid monotherapy. Other studies of particular AEDs have reported that the child's IQ level is negatively correlated with *in utero* exposure to primidone[40], phenobarbital[43] and phenytoin[47].

Microcephaly has been associated with *in utero* AED exposure[9,10]. One multicenter, prospective study found that the risk for small head circumference was increased with polytherapy, phenobarbital and primidone[48].

The risk of epilepsy in children of women with epilepsy is higher (relative risk of 3.2), compared with controls[49]. Children of fathers with epilepsy do not demonstrate this same degree of increased risk. This may be related to the finding that the occurrence of maternal seizures during pregnancy, but not AED use, confers an increased risk of seizures in the offspring (relative risk 2.4)[50].

Mortality

Fetal death (fetal loss at greater than 20 weeks' gestational age) is another increased risk for women with epilepsy. Reported stillbirth rates vary between 1.3 and 14.0% compared with rates of 1.2–7.8% for women without epilepsy[9]. Perinatal death rates are also up to two-fold higher for women with epilepsy (1.3–7.8%), compared with controls (1.0–3.9%)[9]. Spontaneous abortions (< 20 weeks' gestational age) may also occur more frequently, although figures from different studies vary considerably[5,11,51].

Potential mechanisms

The causes of 'anticonvulsant embryopathy' are probably multifactorial. However, recent studies have supported anticonvulsant drugs as being the most significant offending factor, more so than actual traits carried by mothers with epilepsy, environmental factors or possibly even seizures during pregnancy[30,52,53]. A recent research group reported that infants whose mothers had a history of epilepsy but took no AEDs during pregnancy did not have a higher frequency of these abnormalities compared with control infants[52], including abnormalities of cognitive function[53].

Teratogenecity of AEDs is probably mediated by several mechanisms, including antifolate effects and reactive intermediates of AEDs. Phenytoin, carbamazepine, phenobarbital and primidone are associated with folate deficiency, and valproic acid and lamotrigine interfere with folate metabolism[17,54,55]. The beneficial effects of folic acid supplementation are clear for lowering the risk of neural tube defects[56,57]. It may also reduce the risks of other major malformations[58]. The maximal benefit of folate is achieved, however, only with folate supplementation beginning prior to and continuing after conception. Because of this, as well as high rates of unplanned pregnancies and of late contact with a physician, all women with epilepsy of child-bearing potential should be placed on folate supplementation of at least 0.4 mg/day[5]. The American College of Obstetricians and Gynecologists recommends that women with epilepsy who are treated with valproic acid or carbamazepine receive 4 mg/day of folic acid[59].

Reactive intermediates of AEDs include free radicals (via peroxidation reactions) and oxidative metabolites, both of which may contribute to AED teratogenesis[60]. AED polytherapy may especially promote epoxide production and inhibit epoxide metabolism via epoxide hydrolase. Fetuses may benefit from AEDs which lack epoxide intermediates (such as oxcarbazepine, gabapentin) and avoidance of polytherapy.

SEIZURES DURING PREGNANCY

The effect of pregnancy on seizure frequency is variable and unpredictable between patients. According to recent studies, approximately

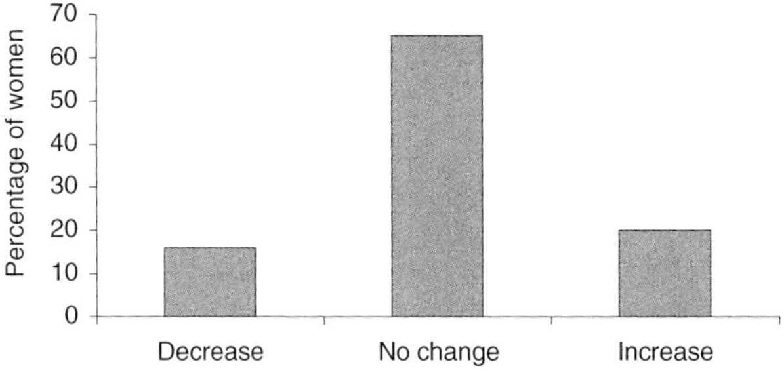

Figure 1 Percentage of women with a change in seizure frequency during pregnancy, compared with preconception baseline

20–33% of patients will have an increase in their seizures, 7–25% a decrease in seizures and 50–83% will experience no significant change[61–64] (Figure 1). The likelihood of seizure worsening cannot be predicted based upon the patient's epilepsy syndrome, type of AED(s) used, seizure type, baseline seizure frequency or even seizure frequency during a previous pregnancy.

Pregnancy is associated with several physiologic and psychologic changes that can alter seizure frequency, including changes in sex hormone concentrations, changes in AED metabolism, sleep deprivation and new stresses. One study demonstrated that sleep deprivation or non-compliance played a clear role in up to 70% of women with an increase in seizures during pregnancy[65], so it is important to enquire about both sleep patterns and compliance in pregnant patients with epilepsy. Sleep deprivation can be due to physical discomforts, movements of the fetus and nocturia. Marital and financial stress and personal doubts and concerns can contribute to sleep deprivation, as well as cause a more direct increase in likelihood of seizure occurrence. Non-compliance with medications is common during pregnancy, and is in large part due to the strong message that any drugs taken during pregnancy are harmful to the fetus. Teratogenic effects of AEDs are well-described, but risks to the fetus are often exaggerated or misrepresented. Proper education about the risks of AEDs versus the risks of seizures can be very helpful in assuring compliance during pregnancy.

During pregnancy, the risk of seizures to the fetus is important, and should be discussed thoroughly with the patient and other family members. Generalized tonic–clonic seizures (GTCSs) can cause maternal and fetal hypoxia and acidosis[9,66]. After a single GTCS, fetal intracranial hemorrhages[67], miscarriages and stillbirths have been reported[17]. A single brief tonic–clonic seizure has been shown to cause depression of the fetal heart rate for more than 20 min[68], and longer or repetitive tonic–clonic seizures are incrementally more hazardous to the fetus as well as the mother. Status epilepticus is an uncommon complication of pregnancy, but when it does occur it carries a high maternal and fetal mortality rate. One series of 29 cases reported nine maternal deaths and 14 infant deaths[69].

It is not as clear what the effects of non-convulsive seizures are on the developing fetus. One study demonstrated that maternal seizures of all types in the first trimester were associated with a higher malformation rate of 12.3%, compared with a malformation rate of 4% for infants of epileptic mothers not exposed to seizures during the first trimester[22]. No significant differences in malformation rates have been observed between offspring of women with different types of epilepsy[20,22]. One case report described that during labor a complex partial seizure was associated with a strong, prolonged uterine contraction with fetal heart rate deceleration for 3.5 min[70]. Many types of seizures can cause trauma, which can result in ruptured fetal membranes with an increased risk of infection, premature labor and even fetal death[16]. Abruptio placentae occurs after 1–5% of minor and 20–50% of major blunt injuries[71]. Restrictions from driving and climbing heights should be reinforced with each patient, with special emphasis on the risk to the fetus of a seemingly minor injury.

In addition to the potential risks of seizures to the developing fetus, re-emergence of seizures in a woman who had previously experienced seizure control can be devastating. Besides the immediate risk to herself and the fetus, she will lose her ability to drive legally, with potential other psychosocial effects.

ANTIEPILEPTIC DRUG MANAGEMENT

Management of AEDs during pregnancy can be complex. Plasma AED concentrations decrease significantly during pregnancy, despite steady or increasing doses, and tend to rise again postpartum[64,72–74]. A similar but even exaggerated effect is seen with lamotrigine[23,72,73,75,76]. Several factors contribute to the decline in AED levels during pregnancy[16]. The most important contributing mechanisms are thought to be decreased albumin concentration with reduced plasma protein binding, and increased drug clearance. The decline in albumin concentration and plasma protein binding creates an increased percentage of unbound AED, which in turn provides an increased proportion of the drug available for metabolic degradation. Additionally, the increased sex steroid hormone levels cause an induction of the hepatic microsomal enzymes and contribute to the increased clearance of AEDs.

The changes in AED levels during pregnancy can vary widely, and are not predictable for the individual based upon reported group changes or total levels only for moderately highly protein-bound AEDs. Although the ratio of free/bound drug increases during pregnancy, the amount of free AED still usually declines[9,64]. The optimal approach to monitoring AED levels during pregnancy is one that measures free levels of any AED that is highly or moderately protein-bound[5]. Total levels are sufficient for AEDs that are minimally protein-bound. The ideal AED (free) level(s) need to be established for each individual patient prior to conception, and should be the level at which seizure control is the best possible for that patient without debilitating side-effects. Levels should be obtained at least at baseline prior to conception and repeated at the beginning of each trimester and again in the last 4 weeks of pregnancy[5]. Some authors recommend monthly monitoring, given the possibility of rapid and unpredictable decreases in AED levels in an individual patient[64,72,75,77]. The frequency of monitoring levels will need to be tailored to each situation, including increased monitoring for worsening seizure control, adverse effects and compliance issues.

OBSTETRIC COMPLICATIONS

Women with epilepsy have an increased risk of certain obstetric complications. There is an approximate two-fold increased risk of vaginal bleeding, anemia, hyperemesis gravidarum, abruptio placentae, eclampsia, premature rupture of the membranes, induced labor and Cesarean section[9]. Weak uterine contractions have been described in women taking AEDs, which may account for the two-fold increased use of interventions during labor and delivery, including induction, mechanical rupture of the membranes, forceps or vacuum assistance and Cesarean sections[78].

NEONATAL VITAMIN K DEFICIENCY

Offspring of women with epilepsy are also at increased risk for a hemorrhagic disorder during the neonatal period, owing to a deficiency of vitamin K-dependent clotting factors[79,80]. One study of 25 women on AEDs found that maternal vitamin K concentrations were lower, and the presence of detectable PIVKA-II (protein induced by vitamin K absence of factor II) in cord samples was higher in the AED group, compared with controls[80]. These abnormalities reversed with the administration of 10 mg of vitamin K_1 daily, beginning at 36 weeks' gestational age[81]. AEDs that have been reported to induce vitamin K deficiency in the fetus include carbamazepine, phenytoin, phenobarbital, ethosuximide, vigabatrin, primidone, diazepam, mephobarbital and amobarbital[9,82]. The mechanism is unclear. Infant mortality from this bleeding disorder is greater than 30%, and is usually due to bleeding in the abdominal and pleural cavities leading to shock. Prophylactic treatment consists of vitamin K_1 administered orally as 10 mg to the mother during the last month of pregnancy, and 1 mg administered intramuscularly or intravenously to the newborn at birth[5]. If the woman has not received supplemental vitamin K_1 prior to labor onset, then she should receive parenteral vitamin K_1. If two of the neonate's coagulation factors fall below 5% of the normal values, intravenous fresh frozen plasma should be administered[11].

LABOR AND DELIVERY

Although there is an approximately two-fold increased use of interventions during labor and delivery[78], most women with epilepsy will have a safe vaginal delivery. GTCSs occur during labor in 1–2% of women with epilepsy, and in another 1–2% during the first 24 h after delivery[31]. Sleep deprivation may provoke seizures, and obstetric anesthesia may be used to allow for some rest prior to delivery if sleep deprivation has been prolonged. During a prolonged labor, oral absorption of AEDs may be erratic, and any emesis will confound the problem. Phenobarbital, (fos)phenytoin and valproic acid can be given intravenously at the same maintenance dosage. Convulsive seizures and repeated seizures during labor should be treated promptly with parenteral lorazepam or Valium®[31]. Benzodiazepines can cause neonatal depression, decreased heart rate and maternal apnea if given in large doses, and these potential side-effects need to be monitored closely. Administration of another, longer-acting AED is controversial owing to the inhibitory effects on myometrial contractions[31].

Status epilepticus, or even a single GTCS, needs to be treated aggressively because of the high risk to the mother and fetus. Oxygen should be administered to the patient and she should be placed on her left side to increase uterine blood flow and decrease the risk of maternal aspiration[38]. Prompt Cesarean section should be performed when repeated GTCSs cannot be controlled during labor, or when the mother is unable to co-operate during labor because of impaired awareness during repetitive absence or complex partial seizures[31]. The analgesic meperidine is best avoided because of its potential to lower seizure threshold.

POSTPARTUM CARE

Serum antiepileptic drug levels rise again after delivery and plateau after 8–10 weeks. AED levels should be followed closely during this postpartum period[5].

Table 3 Breast milk/maternal plasma ratio of common antiepileptic drugs[83]

Carbamazepine	0.69
Phenytoin	0.45
Phenobarbital	0.4–0.6
Primidone	0.72
Valproic acid	0.42
Lamotrigine	0.6

Perinatal lethargy, irritability and feeding difficulties have been attributed to intrauterine exposure to barbiturates and benzodiazepines, and breast-feeding with barbiturates or benzodiazepines may prolong sedation and feeding problems. However, most infants of women with epilepsy can successfully breast-feed without complications, especially if the infant is monitored closely. Concentrations of the different AEDs in breast milk are considerably less than those in maternal serum (Table 3). The infant's serum concentration is determined by this factor as well as the AED elimination half-life in neonates, which is usually more prolonged than that in adults[11,84]. The benefits of breast-feeding are believed to outweigh the small risk of adverse effects of AEDs[5,36].

The puerperium along with its inevitable sleep disruption is often a time of seizure worsening, and may even provoke seizure recurrence for women with previously controlled seizures. Extra precautions should be taken during this time[85]. Appropriate individualized safety issues must consider the mother's ictal semiology. If she is likely to drop objects she is holding but remain upright, such as with myoclonic seizures or many complex partial seizures, then she should use a harness when carrying the baby. If she is likely to fall, then a stroller within the house is an even better option. Changing diapers and clothes is best done on the floor rather than on an elevated changing table. Bathing should never be performed alone, as a brief lapse in attention can result in a fatal drowning. The important role that sleep deprivation plays in exacerbation of seizures needs to be emphasized. Especially if the mother is breast-feeding, sleep deprivation may be unavoidable. The possibility of other adults sharing the burden of night-time feeds through the use of formula or harvested breast milk should be considered, and the mother should attempt to make up any missed sleep during the infant's daytime naps.

SUMMARY OF MANAGEMENT OF EPILEPSY AND PREGNANCY

Comprehensive care of women with epilepsy during the reproductive years must include effective preconceptional counseling. This includes discussions about birth control and the lower efficacy of many hormonal contraceptive agents with the hepatic enzyme-inducing AEDs. The woman's AED regimen should be optimized, and folate supplementation should be begun prior to pregnancy. Although AEDs carry teratogenic risks, for most women with epilepsy withdrawal of all AEDs prior to pregnancy is not a realistic option. A decision to undergo a trial off AEDs prior to a planned pregnancy should be based upon the same principles used for AED withdrawal in any person with epilepsy[86]. The taper should be completed at least 6 months prior to planned conception to provide some reassurance that seizures are not going to recur[5]. If a woman with epilepsy is in the more prevalent category of needing AEDs for seizure control, then monotherapy at the lowest effective dose should be employed. If large daily doses are needed, then frequent smaller doses or extended-release formulations may be helpful to avoid high peak levels.

A common but erroneous reason to change medications is the woman who presents to the neurologist after she has discovered she is pregnant. In many cases, she is already in or past the critical period of organogenesis (Table 4). If a woman with epilepsy presents after conception who is taking a single AED that is effective, her medication should usually not be changed. Exposing the fetus to a second agent during a cross-over period of AEDs only increases the teratogenic risk, and seizures are more likely to occur with any abrupt medication change. If a woman is on polytherapy and seizure-free, then it may be possible to switch safely to monotherapy. However, changes in the total and free levels of the remaining drug will need to be monitored closely.

Seizure control remains an important goal during pregnancy. Convulsive seizures in particular place the mother and fetus at risk. Nonconvulsive seizures may also be harmful, especially if they involve falling or other forms of trauma. Since each of the major AEDs is teratogenic, the medication that is most effective for that woman's epilepsy and seizure type should be prescribed.

Folate supplementation should begin prior to conception and is crucial during the first 30 days of gestation to protect against neural

Table 4 Relative timing and developmental pathology of certain malformations[87]

Tissues	*Malformation*	*Post-conceptional age* (days)
CNS	neural tube defect	28
Heart	ventricular septal defect	42
Face	cleft lip	36
	cleft maxillary palate	70

CNS, central nervous system

tube defects. The optimal dosage has not been established for women on AEDs, and recommendations vary between 0.4 and 5 mg/day.

Prenatal screening can detect major malformations in the first and second trimesters. Vitamin K_1 is given as 10 mg/day orally during the last month of pregnancy, followed by 1 mg intramuscularly or intravenously to the newborn[5].

With the above information and guidelines, most women with epilepsy will have healthy pregnancies without major maternal or fetal complications.

References

1. Holmes LB. The teratogenecity of anticonvulsant drugs: a progress report. *J Med Genet* 2002;39:245–7
2. Fairgrieve SD, Jackson M, Jonas P, *et al.* Population based, prospective study of the care of women with epilepsy in pregnancy. *Br Med J* 2000; 321:674–5
3. Janz D, Schmidt D. Anti-epileptic drugs and failure of oral contraceptives. *Lancet* 1974;1:113
4. Guberman A. Hormonal contraception and epilepsy. *Neurology* 1999; 53(Suppl 1):S38–40
5. Report of the Quality Standards Subcommittee of the American Academy of Neurology. Practice parameter: management issues for women with epilepsy (summary statement). *Neurology* 1998;51:944–8
6. Krauss G, Brandt J, Campbell M, *et al.* Antiepileptic medication and oral contraceptive interactions: a national survey of neurologists and obstetricians. *Neurology* 1996;46:1534–9
7. Rosenfeld W, Doose D, Walker S, *et al.* Effect of topiramate on the pharmacokinetics of an oral contraceptive containing norethindrone and ethinyl estradiol in patients with epilepsy. *Epilepsia* 1997;38:317–23
8. Shane-McWhorter L, Cerveny J, MacFarlane L, *et al.* Enhanced metabolism of levonorgestrel during phenobarbital treatment and resultant pregnancy. *Pharmacotherapy* 1998;18:1360–4
9. Yerby MS. Quality of life, epilepsy advances, and the evolving role of anticonvulsants in women with epilepsy. *Neurology* 2000;55(Suppl 5): S21–31, discussion S54–8
10. Hvas C, Henriksen T, Ostergaard J, *et al.* Epilepsy and pregnancy: effect of antiepileptic drugs and lifestyle on birthweight. *Br J Obstet Gynaecol* 2000;107:896–902
11. Yerby M, Collins S. Teratogenecity of antiepileptic drugs. In Engel J, Pedley T, eds. *Epilepsy, a Comprehensive Textbook.* Philadelphia: Lippincott-Raven, 1997:1195–203
12. Gilmore J, Pennell PB, Stern BJ. Medication use during pregnancy for neurologic conditions. In Evans R, ed. *Neurologic Clinics: Iatrogenic Disorders.* Philadelphia: WB Saunders, 1998:189–206
13. Arpino C, Brescianini S, Robert E, *et al.* Teratogenic effects of antiepileptic drugs: use of an international database on malformations and drug exposure (MADRE). *Epilepsia* 2000;41:1436–43

14. Wide K, Winbladh B, Tomson T, *et al*. Body dimensions of infants exposed to antiepileptic drugs *in utero*: observations spanning 25 years. *Epilepsia* 2000;41:854–61
15. Morrell M. Guidelines for the care of women with epilepsy. *Neurology* 1998;51(Suppl 5):S21–7
16. Yerby M, Devinsky O. Epilepsy and pregnancy. In Devinsky O, Feldmann E, Hainline B, eds. *Advances in Neurology: Neurological Complications of Pregnancy*. New York: Raven Press, 1994:45–63
17. Zahn CA, Morrell MJ, Collins SD, *et al*. Management issues for women with epilepsy: a review of the literature. *Neurology* 1998;51:949–56
18. Kaneko S, Battino D, Andermann E, *et al*. Congenital malformations due to antiepileptic drugs. *Epilepsy Res* 1999;33:145–58
19. Lindhout D, Omtzigt J, Cornel M. Spectrum of neural-tube defects in 34 infants perinatally exposed to antiepileptic drugs. *Neurology* 1992; 42(Suppl 5):111–18
20. Samrén E, van Duijn C, Koch S, *et al*. Maternal use of antiepileptic drugs and the risk of major congenital malformations: a joint European prospective study of human teratogenesis asssociated with maternal epilepsy. *Epilepsia* 1997;38:981–90
21. Dean J, Hailey H, Moore S, *et al*. Long term health and neurodevelopment in children exposed to antiepileptic drugs before birth. *J Med Genet* 2002;39:251–9
22. Lindhout D, Meinardi H, Meijer J, *et al*. Antiepileptic drugs and teratogenesis in two consecutive cohorts: changes in prescription policy paralleled by changes in pattern of malformations. *Neurology* 1992;42(Suppl 5):94–110
23. Kaneko S, Otani K, Fukushima Y, *et al*. Malformations in infants of mothers with epilepsy receiving antiepileptic drugs. *Neurology* 1992;42(Suppl 5):68–74
24. Oguni M, Dansky L, Andermann E, *et al*. Improved pregnancy outcome in epileptic women in the last decade: relationship to maternal anticonvulsant therapy [Comment]. *Brain Dev* 1992;14:371–80
25. Kaneko S, Otani K, Fukushima Y. Teratogenicity of antiepileptic drugs: analysis of possible risk factors. *Epilepsia* 1988;29:459–67
26. Samrén E, van Duijn C, Christiaens G, *et al*. Antiepileptic drug regimens and major congenital abnormalities in the offspring. *Ann Neurol* 1999; 46:739–46
27. Dravet C, Julian C, Legras C, *et al*. Epilepsy, antiepileptic drugs, and malformations in children of women with epilepsy: a French prospective cohort study. *Neurology* 1992;42(Suppl 5):75–82
28. Rosa F. Spina bifida in infants of women treated with carbamazepine during pregnancy. *N Engl J Med* 1991;324:674–7
29. Lindhout D, Schmidt D. *In-utero* exposure to valproate and neural tube defects. *Lancet* 1986;2:1392–3
30. Canger R, Battino D, Canerini M, *et al*. Malformations in offspring of women with epilepsy: a prospective study. *Epilepsia* 1999;40:1231–6
31. Delgado-Escueta A, Janz D. Consensus guidelines: preconception counseling, management, and care of the pregnant woman with epilepsy. *Neurology* 1992;42:149–60

32. Holmes L, Lieberman E. Report of first positive findings from hospital-based AED pregnancy registry. *Teratology* 2001;63:250
33. Holmes L, Wyszynski D, Mittendorf R. Evidence for an increased risk of birth defects in the offspring of women exposed to valproate: findings from the AED pregnancy registry. *Am J Obstet Gynecol* 2002;187:5137
34. Holmes L. *The North American AED Pregnancy Registry*. Charlestown, MA: Harvard Medical School, 2003
35. *Lamotrogine. Lamotrogine pregnancy registry, interim report, 9/1/92–3/31/02*. Research Triangle Park, NC: GlaxoSmithKline, 2002
36. Pschirrer E, Monga M. Seizure disorders in pregnancy. *Obstet Gynecol Clin* 2001;28:601–11
37. Malone F, D'Alton M. Drugs in pregnancy: anticonvulsants. *Semin Perinatol* 1997;21:114–23
38. Committee on Educational Bulletins of the American College of Obstetricians and Gynecologists. Seizure disorders in pregnancy. *Int J Gynecol Obstet* 1997;56:279–86
39. Ganström M, Gaily E. Psychomotor development in children of mothers with epilepsy. *Neurology* 1992;42(Suppl 5):144–8
40. Koch S, Titze K, Zimmerman R, *et al*. Long-term neuropsychological consequences of maternal epilepsy and anticonvulsant treatment during pregnancy for school-age children and adolescents. *Epilepsia* 1999;40: 1237–43
41. Adab N, Jacoby A, Smith D, *et al*. Additional educational needs in children born to mothers with epilepsy. *J Neurol Neurosurg Psychiatry* 2001; 70:15–21
42. Matalon S, Schechtman S, Goldzweig G, *et al*. The teratogenic effect of carbamazepine: a meta-analysis of 1255 exposures. *Reprod Toxicol* 2002; 16:9–17
43. Reinisch J, Sanders S, Mortensen E, *et al*. *In utero* exposure to phenobarbital and intelligence deficits in adult men. *J Am Med Assoc* 1995;724: 1518–25
44. Leavitt A, Yerby M, Robinson N, *et al*. Epilepsy in pregnancy: developmental outcome of offspring at 12 months. *Neurology* 1992;42(Suppl 5): 141–3
45. Leonard G, Andermann E, Ptito A. Cognitive effects of antiepileptic drug therapy during pregnancy on school-age offspring [Abstract]. *Epilepsia* 1997;38(Suppl 3):170
46. Meador K. Cognitive effects of epilepsy and of antiepileptic medications. In Wyllie E, ed. *The Treatment of Epilepsy: Principles and Practice*, 3rd edn. Philadelphia: Williams & Wilkins, 2001:1215–26
47. Vanoverloop D, Schnell R, Harvey E, *et al*. The effects of prenatal exposure to phenytoin and other anticonvulsants on intellectual function at 4 to 8 years of age. *Neurotoxicol Teratol* 1992;14:329–35
48. Battino D, Kaneko S, Andermann E, *et al*. Intrauterine growth in the offspring of epileptic women: a prospective multicenter study. *Epilepsy Res* 1999;36:53–60
49. Annegers J, Hauser W, Elveback L, *et al*. Congenital malformations and seizure disorders in the offspring of parents with epilepsy. *Int J Epidemiol* 1978;7:241–7

50. Ottman R, Annegers J, Hauser W, *et al.* Higher risk of seizures in offspring of mothers than fathers with epilepsy. *Am J Hum Genet* 1988;43: 357–64
51. Yerby M, Cawthon M. Fetal death, malformations and infant mortality in infants of mothers with epilepsy. *Epilepsia* 1996;37(Suppl 5):98
52. Holmes LB, Harvey EA, Coull BA, *et al.* The teratogenicity of anticonvulsant drugs. *N Engl J Med* 2001;344:1132–8
53. Holmes LB, Rosenberger PB, Harvey EA, Intelligence and physical features of children of women with epilepsy. *Teratology* 2000;61:196–202
54. Dansky L, Rosenblatt D, Andermann E. Mechanisms of teratogenesis: folic acid and antiepileptic therapy. *Neurology* 1992;42:32–42
55. Wegner C, Nau H. Alteration of embryonic folate metabolism by valproic acid during organogenesis: implications for mechanisms of teratogenesis. *Neurology* 1992;42(Suppl 5):17–24
56. Botto L, Moore C, Khoury M, *et al.* Medical progress: neural-tube defects. *N Engl J Med* 1999;341:1509–19
57. MRC Vitamin Study Research Group. Prevention of neural-tube defects: results of the Medical Research Council Vitamin Study. *Lancet* 1991;338: 131–7
58. Hall J, Solehdin F. Folic acid for the prevention of congential anomalies. *Eur J Pediatr* 1998;157:445–50
59. Crawford P. CPD-education and self-assessment: epilepsy and pregnancy. *Seizure* 2001;10:212–19
60. Buehler BA, Rao V, Finnell RH. Biochemical and molecular teratology of fetal hydantoin syndrome. *Pediatr Neurogenet* 1994;12:741–8
61. Devinsky O, Yerby M. Women with epilepsy. *Neurol Clin* 1994;12:479–95
62. Pennell P. Pregnancy in the woman with epilepsy: maternal and fetal outcomes. *Semin Neurol* 2002;22:299–307
63. Cantrell D. Epilepsy and pregnancy: a study of seizure frequency and patient demographics. *Epilepsia* 1997;38(Suppl 8):231
64. Yerby M, Collins S. Pregnancy and the mother. In Engel J, Pedley T, eds. *Epilepsy, a Comprehensive Textbook*. Philadelphia: Lippincott-Raven, 1997: 2027–35
65. Schmidt D, Canger R, Avanzini G, *et al.* Change of seizure frequency in pregnant epileptic women. *J Neurol Neurosurg Psychiatry* 1983;46:751–5
66. Stumpf D, Frost M. Seizures, anticonvulsants, and pregnancy. *Am J Dis Child* 1978;132:746–8
67. Minkoff H, Schaffer R, Delke I, *et al.* Diagnosis of intracranial hemorrhage *in utero* after a maternal seizure. *Obstet Gynecol* 1985;65(Suppl): 22S–24S
68. Teramo K, Hiilesmaa V, Bardy A, *et al.* Fetal heart rate during a maternal grand mal epileptic seizure. *J Perinat Med* 1979;7:3–5
69. Teramo K, Hiilesmaa V. Pregnancy and fetal complications in epileptic pregnancies: review of the literature. In Janz D, Bossi L, Dam M, *et al.*, eds. *Epilepsy, Pregnancy and the Child.* New York: Raven Press, 1982:53–9
70. Nei M, Daly S, Liporace J. A maternal complex partial seizure in labor can affect fetal heart rate. *Neurology* 1998;51:904–6
71. Pearlman M, Tintinalli J, Lorenz R. Blunt trauma during pregnancy. *N Engl J Med* 1990;323:1609–13

72. Pennell P, Gleba J, Clements S. Antiepileptic drug monitoring during pregnancy in women with epilepsy. *Epilepsia* 2000;41(Suppl 7):200
73. Ohman I, Vitols S, Tomson T. Lamotrigine in pregnancy: pharmacokinetics during delivery, in the neonate and during lactation. *Epilepsia* 2000;41:709–13
74. Yerby MS. The use of anticonvulsants during pregnancy. *Semin Perinatol* 2001;25:153–8
75. Pennell P, Montgomery J, Clements S, Newport D. Lamotrigine clearance markedly increases during pregnancy. *Epilepsia* 2002;43(Suppl 7): 234
76. Sathanandar S, Blesi K, Tran T, *et al*. Lamotrigine clearance increases markedly during pregnancy. *Epilepsia* 2000;41(Suppl 7):246
77. Levy R, Yerby M. Effects of pregnancy on antiepileptic drug utilization. *Epilepsia* 1985;26(Suppl 1):S52–7
78. Yerby M, Koepsell T, Daling J. Pregnancy complications and outcomes in a cohort of women with epilepsy. *Epilepsia* 1985;26:631–5
79. Howe A, Oakes D, Woodman P, *et al*. Prothrombin and PIVKA-II levels in cord blood from newborn exposed to anticonvulsants during pregnancy. *Epilepsia* 1999;40:980–4
80. Cornellisen M, Steegers-Theunissen R, Kollee L, *et al*. Increased incidence of neonatal vitamin K deficiency resulting from maternal anticonvulsant therapy. *Am J Obstet Gynecol* 1993;168:923–8
81. Cornellisen M, Steegers-Theunissen R, Kollee L, *et al*. Supplementation of vitamin K in pregnant women receiving anticonvulsant therapy prevents neonatal vitamin K deficiency. *Am J Obstet Gynecol* 1993;168:884–8
82. Srinivasan G, Seeler RA, Tiruvury A, *et al*. Maternal anticonvulsant therapy and hemorrhagic disease of the newborn. *Obstet Gynecol* 1982;59: 250–2
83. Hale T. *Medications and Mothers' Milk*, 8th edn. Amarillo: Pharmasoft Medical Publishing, 1999
84. Krauer B, Krauer F. Drug kinetics in pregnancy. *Clin Pharmacokinet* 1977; 2:167–81
85. Fox C, Betts T. How much risk does a woman with active epilepsy pose to her newborn child in the puerperium? A pilot study. *Seizure* 1999;86: 367–9
86. Report of the Quality Standards Subcommittee of the American Academy of Neurology. Practice parameter: a guideline for discontinuing antiepileptic drugs in seizure-free patients – summary statement. *Neurology* 1996;47:600–2
87. Moore K. *The Developing Human: Clinically Oriented Embryology*, 4th edn. Philadelphia: WB Saunders, 1988

4

Back pain

J. M. Gilchrist

INTRODUCTION

Low back pain is a frequent accompaniment to pregnancy, at least in part due to many unique changes occurring during pregnancy, several of which affect the lumbosacral and pelvic regions. Low back and pelvic pain can also complicate delivery, and contribute to disability after delivery.

ANATOMY AND BIOMECHANICS

The lower back is a poorly understood machine, imperfectly designed for the task of bipedal transportation, and required to be supportive, protective and flexible. The bony vertebral column can be divided into two parts: the anterior, consisting of the vertebral bodies and the intervertebral disks, and the posterior, consisting of the pedicles, the facets and the spinous processes. The duties of the anterior portion include weight-bearing (which in the lumbar spine includes most of the body's weight) and shock absorption. The posterior portion is not weight-bearing, and has been described as the 'gliding, guiding'[1] mechanism of the spine, also providing protection for the neural elements, the spinal cord and the nerve roots.

Integrating with the vertebral column are several other important, and pain-sensitive, structures and tissues including blood vessels, nerves, ligaments, tendons, periosteum, fascia, muscles and meninges. The end result is a column with three curves: a cervical and a lumbar lordosis, and a thoracic kyphosis. The center of gravity at the caudal lumbar level is actually anterior to the vertebral bodies, necessitating a compensatory anterior tilt of the vertebral column, and creating increased shear on the intervertebral disks which must be counterbalanced by ligaments and muscles[2].

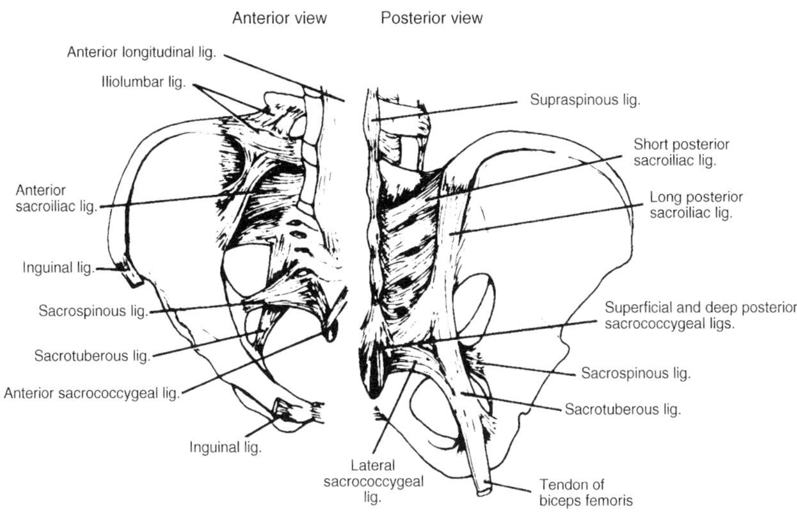

Figure 1 Anterior and posterior views of the sacroiliac joint ligaments. Reproduced with permission from reference 3

The spine ends in the sacrum, which consists of five fused vertebral bodies without intervertebral disks. The sacrum connects to the pelvis via the sacroiliac joints. Extensive ligamental connections hold this joint together (Figure 1). Anteriorly, the halves of the pelvis are connected at the symphysis pubis by short, sturdy ligamentous connections.

EFFECT OF PREGNANCY UPON THE LOWER BACK AND PELVIS

Several changes occurring during pregnancy may be pertinent in the production of low back pain. An obvious change is the increased body weight in general, and in the abdomen in particular. The gravid uterus creates a prominent anterior protuberance which has been presumed to shift the center of gravity anteriorly, resulting in the pelvis tilting downwards, increasing lumbar lordosis and increasing stress on the vertebral elements[1]. This is controversial, with some authors concluding that in fact the entire vertebral column straightens and shifts backwards, with a posterior movement of the center of gravity and no increase in lumbar lordosis[4].

The large abdomen stretches the abdominal musculature, which is an important element in back support, causing decreased tone and increased strain on vertebral elements. Ligamentous relaxation also occurs, involving the powerful sacroiliac ligaments bilaterally, well described in the literature since Abrahamson and colleagues[5] in 1934 and Young[6] in 1940. This relaxation is largely from the effects of the hormone relaxin, which increases ten-fold during pregnancy[7]. Joint laxity also occurs, most notably involving the symphysis pubis, first described in 1899[8], which may widen by more than a centimeter[9], also related to increases in relaxin during pregnancy. This widening causes increased rotatory stress on the sacroiliac joints, which is exacerbated by the conjoint laxity of sacroiliac ligaments. The pelvis becomes increasingly unstable as the three pelvic joints loosen, which is a necessity for normal delivery, but which turns walking, lifting and rotation of the pelvis into painful endeavors.

Intravascular volume increases in pregnancy, and as the uterus enlarges it can compromise the inferior vena cava, especially when the woman is recumbent. These two factors can lead to venous engorgement caudal to the compression, including pelvic veins and the vertebral venous plexus, with resultant edema and stasis of the vasa nervosum of nerve roots[10]. This tends to be worse when the woman is recumbent, such as at night. It is unlikely that the enlarged uterus rotating posteriorly and directly compressing nerve roots is a factor, given the intervening muscles, vertebral bodies and disks, although a case of lumbosacral plexus compression has been reported[11].

TYPES OF LOW BACK PAIN AND THEIR INCIDENCE

Low back pain is very common during pregnancy, a fact known since ancient times and documented by several retrospective and prospective studies in the past 25 years[12–21] (Table 1). But low back pain during pregnancy is not a unitary concept, as pregnant women suffer a variety of pain syndromes, including lumbar pain, pelvic girdle pain, nighttime back pain and back pain during labor. Virtually all studies have found that more than half of all women will complain of low back pain at some point during pregnancy[12–16]. Mantle and colleagues[12] surveyed 180 women at the time of delivery and found that 48% experienced back pain, and one-third described it as severe. A decade later, Fast and associates[14] interviewed 200 women shortly after delivery and 56% complained of back pain, just under half of whom had radiation of the pain to their legs. Berg and co-workers[15] in 1988 performed the first prospective survey of back pain during pregnancy, and confirmed that at least 50% were afflicted. They were the first to recognize that the majority of pregnancy patients have posterior pelvic pain, as opposed to lumbar pain, at the site of their low back pain. Since then, several prospective studies have verified the existence of posterior pelvic pain as a separate syndrome from lumbar pain, and have confirmed that the incidence of posterior pelvic pain is more common than that of lumbar pain[17–20]. Ostgaard and colleagues[17] followed 368 women from mid-

Table 1 Summary of studies of the incidence of low back and posterior pelvic pain during pregnancy

Authors	*Year*	*Type*	*n*	*Percentage with pain*
Low back pain (including pelvic pain)				
Mantle *et al.*[12]	1977	retrospective	180	60
Heckman and Sassard[13]	1994	retrospective	126	70
Fast *et al.*[14]	1987	retrospective	200	56
Berg *et al.*[15]	1988	prospective	862	49
Orvieto *et al.*[16]	1994	prospective	246	55
Ostgaard *et al.*[17]	1996	prospective	368	45
Sturesson *et al.*[18]	1997	prospective	335	51
Noren *et al.*[21]	2002	prospective	799	29
Posterior pelvic pain				
Ostgaard *et al.*[17]	1996	prospective	368	34
Sturesson *et al.*[18]	1997	prospective	335	36
Larsen *et al.*[19]	1999	prospective	1600	14
Albert *et al.*[20]	2000	prospective	2269	24

pregnancy until 5 months after delivery, and during pregnancy 34% had posterior pelvic pain, while only 11% had lumbar pain. However, after delivery, back pain was the more common complaint. Sturesson and colleagues[18] found that 51% of their pregnant patients had low back pain, 71% of whom had signs at examination indicative of a posterior pelvic source for their pain. Larsen and co-workers[19] surveyed 1600 consecutive women for posterior pelvic pain throughout their pregnancy and for 1 year after delivery. The incidence during pregnancy was 14%, which dropped after delivery to 5% at 2 months, 4% at 6 months and 2% by 1 year. Finally, Albert and associates[20] questioned and examined 2269 consecutive pregnant women, and found that 535 (24%) had complaints of daily pelvic pain and signs of pelvic joint dysfunction.

Following the acknowledgement that posterior pelvic pain was common during pregnancy was the recognition that there were various syndromes of pelvic pain. Berg and colleagues[15] studied 79 pregnant women with back pain too severe to allow continued work, and who were extensively examined by an orthopedic surgeon. The most common source of posterior pelvic pain was sacroiliac joint dysfunction, found in two-thirds of the women, frequently accompanied by symphysiolysis. Mild non-specific back pain, symphysiolysis without sacroiliac joint dysfunction, sciatic nerve involvement, thoracic pain and lumbago were the diagnoses in the other women. Albert and associates[22] found a similar distribution of causes of posterior pelvic pain, with 30% of the affected women having pelvic girdle syndrome (i.e. daily pain in all three pelvic joints), 10% having symphysiolysis and 60% suffering either unilateral or bilateral sacroiliac syndrome. Posterior pelvic pain and lumbar pain occur together in up to 40% of women with low back pain[23].

Several authors have related the etiology of posterior pelvic pain to sacroiliac joint dysfunction, correlating symptoms, signs and hormonal levels to the degree and location of pain[20,24]. A prospective study by Kristiansson and colleagues[24] comparing relaxin levels to gestational age and to location of pain found significant correlation with relaxin levels at the 36th week, and with symptoms and signs of pain in the trochanteric and symphysis areas, but not with lumbar spine or low back pain. Relaxin levels increased until reaching a peak value at around 12 weeks of gestation, thereafter they decreased 50% by week 17 and then remained steady until postpartum[24]. The study found a tight correlation between levels of relaxin at various gestation times, indicating that some women had high levels throughout while others had low levels throughout pregnancy[24]. Those women with high levels appeared to be at particular risk for developing posterior pelvic pain. Relaxin levels were non-detectable by 3 months after delivery[24], consistent with the overall good prognosis, particularly of pelvic pain, after delivery.

A much less-recognized syndrome is night backache of pregnancy, which was found in 67% of women during the second half of pregnancy in one study[10], in half of whom it was severe enough to awaken them from sleep. Not uncommonly, nocturnal backache is accompanied by nocturnal cramps. Evening-related worsening is not unexpected as the result of cumulative biomechanical stresses over the day, exacerbated by fatigue. However, this would not as easily explain night-time pain, which can be so severe as to awaken patients. Fast and co-workers[10] hypothesized 'that hypervolemia combined with obstruction of the inferior vena cava, caused by the enlarging uterus' is the underlying cause, leading to 'excessive pressure within the venous system' and hypoxemia, edema and stasis within the spinal nerves, resulting in pain. Intravenous dihydroergotamine, a potent vasoconstrictor, has been used to relieve pelvic venous congestion, and subsequently relieve pain, in menstruating women, providing some support for this theory[25].

Pain is unavoidable during the non-anesthetized delivery, although its severity and location may vary. Melzack and Schaffelberg[26] characterized five types of labor pain: front contractions, back contractions, continuous back pain, perineal pain related to tearing of tissues in the second stage of labor and episiotomy pain. Low back pain, while not as common as abdominal pain, is present in three-quarters of women, with continuous back pain being the worst pain of labor in one-third of women. Many women may be prepared by birthing classes for the contraction pain, but are often taken by surprise by the unremitting back pain. Possible causes include traction on the adnexa, bladder, urethra, rectum and lumbosacral plexus (all of which are pain-sensitive) with pain referred to the low back, reflex muscular spasm in muscles supplied by the same spinal segments as those organs[26] or acute worsening of venous compression and stasis from markedly increased intra-abdominal pressure[2].

EXAMINATION AND CHARACTERISTICS

In general, low back pain and posterior pelvic pain can be differentiated based on the location and nature of the patient's complaints[21]. Low back pain is centered in the lower lumbar area and often does not radiate. The patients will often be tender to palpation in the lower lumbar area and will sometimes have paraspinal muscle spasm. Straight leg raising may elicit pain at acute angles, and pain in the lumbar region will often increase with rotatory or lateral movements. The pain is usually constant, but walking and standing are not likely to worsen discomfort[21]. Posterior pelvic pain is lower and more lateral, usually in the buttocks and radiating to the legs (thighs usually, and rarely to the feet) in 45–65% of patients, with pain-free intervals although frequently worse in the evening or at night, and with activities such as standing, walking, lifting and bending forwards. It is usually a new type of pain, not present before pregnancy.

Sacroiliac joint dysfunction is relatively easy to discern at the bedside[27–29] (Table 2). The active straight leg test has been shown to correlate well with pelvic pain symptoms, radiation of pain and back pain indices, and is a simple way to assess severity of the back pain[30]. Lasegue's test of passive straight leg raising has been helpful in that it is negative in sacroiliac joint dysfunction[15,20], but is often abnormal in lumbar pain syndromes. The femoral compression test, or posterior pelvic pain provocation test[31], is done with the patient supine, with the hip and knee each flexed to 90°. The knee is pushed down into the bed, eliciting pain in the ipsilateral posterior pelvis. Patrick's test is also done with the patient supine, applying pressure to the medial knee while the hip is flexed and abducted, and the knee bent so that the heel rests on the opposite knee. This will cause pain in the ipsilateral abnormal sacroiliac joint. Alternatively, the examiner can cross arms and apply force simultaneously and bilaterally to the inner aspects of the anterior iliac spine, with pain posteriorly on the side of the affected sacroiliac joint (iliac separation or gapping test) or apply force to the outer iliac spines, compressing the pelvis (iliac compression test), again causing pain posteriorly over the sacroiliac joint(s). In trained hands, the iliac separation and compression tests are associated with high interexaminer reliability[20,27,29]. The pelvis may also show posterior asymmetry and abnormal movement during hip flexion. Derbolowski's test is done by

Table 2 Sensitivity of various bedside tests in pregnant women with posterior pelvic pain and sacroiliac joint instability

Test maneuver	*Sacroiliac joint dysfunction* (% positive)	*Pelvic girdle syndrome* (% positive)
Active straight leg raise	94[32]	
Derbolowski's test	19[15]	
Iliac compression	83[15]; 38[20]	70[20]
Iliac separation	87[15]; 14[20]	40[20]
Lasegue, either side	0[15]	
Long dorsal sacroiliac ligament palpation	76[32]; 11[20]; 77[30]	49[20]
Patrick's test	52[15]; 40[20]	70[20]
Posterior pain provocation	81[31]; 93[20]; 69[30]; 76[32]	90[20]
Sacroiliac joint fixation test	33[15]; 21[20]	14[20]

noting the position of the medial malleoli in relation to each other with the patient lying down and then sitting. A shortening of one leg when sitting up indicates an ipsilateral pelvic dysfunction[15]. The sacroiliac joint fixation test assesses the position of the posterior superior spine after flexion of the knee and hip: failure of it to drop during the maneuver indicates reduced sacroiliac joint mobility on that side[15]. Pain on direct palpation of the long dorsal sacroiliac ligament is also a sensitive indicator of posterior pelvic pain[32] (Figure 1). Many of these provocative tests are more useful for reaching a diagnosis of sacroiliac joint dysfunction and less useful for following the patient over time. Internal rotation of the hip has been shown in one prospective study to be the easiest and most reliable bedside test for ongoing pain assessment[33].

The incidence and severity of both low back and posterior pelvic pain tend to increase with gestational age, reaching a peak in the seventh or eighth month. Several investigators have attempted to determine what other factors predispose or protect from pregnancy-related back and pelvic pain, starting with Mantle and colleagues[12] in 1977, who found that back pain increased with increasing maternal age and parity. Unfortunately, this has become rather messy, as several other authors have reached a variety of conclusions about predictive characteristics. Factors clearly not associated with back pain include maternal and fetal weight[10,12,16,34]. Other factors sometimes correlated with back pain, and sometimes not, include maternal age, parity and the presence of back pain before pregnancy[10,16,19,34]. Low back or pelvic pain in previous pregnancies appears to be a reliable predictor of pain in subsequent pregnancies[35]. Low back pain persisting into the postpartum period is common, but it is uncommon to persist longer than 6 months unless there was back pain preceding pregnancy[35]. The incidence of low back pain during pregnancy appears to be less in those women given antenatal back training[36].

DIFFERENT DIAGNOSIS

It would be a reasonable assumption, given the shifting mechanical and physiologic forces increasing the stress and shear upon the vertebral column, that herniated lumbar disks play a major role in causing low back pain during pregnancy. However, there are few data to support that. LaBan and co-workers[37,38] found an incidence of acute lumbar herniated disk of only 1 : 10 000 among their population, and a magnetic resonance imaging study comparing pregnant women with their non-pregnant counterparts found no difference in the incidence of intervertebral disk abnormalities between the two groups[39]. An epidemiologic study found an association between the number of pregnancies resulting in live births and the presence of eventual acute lumbosacral disk herniation (but true only for L5 disks), but was flawed by procedural and diagnostic limitations[40]. In the general population, acute radiculopathy is a relatively uncommon (10%) source of acute back pain, and pregnancy does not appear to change that[41].

Less common causes (some quite rare) of low back pain during pregnancy include degenerative spine disease, spondylolisthesis, spondylolysis, sciatic nerve or lumbosacral plexus compression[11], shingles, sacroiliitis[42], osteomyelitis, neurofibromas and spinal tumors. Of related interest, epidural anesthesia does not appear to predispose to postpartum back pain[43].

PROGNOSIS AND MANAGEMENT

Clearly, one aspect of pregnancy-associated low back pain is universally reversible: pregnancy. Taken with the relative youth of the patients, the prognosis is generally good[21,35,44]. Symptoms can persist for weeks to months after delivery, because the conditions predisposing to back pain also persist for some time after delivery, such as ligamentous laxity, postural changes and diminished muscle tone, with the added stress of inadequate sleep, and lifting and carrying the infant. However, it is uncommon for back pain to persist for longer than 6 months after delivery unless the woman had back pain preceding pregnancy. Prepregnancy back pain, very severe back pain and combined low back and posterior pelvic pain during pregnancy are factors predictive of persistent back pain[21,35,44]. In a prospective, consecutive 3-year cohort study of women who had back pain during pregnancy, Noren and colleagues[21] surveyed 231 women and examined 41 (18%) with persistent pain. Only eight women (3%) had combined lumbar and pelvic pain, but they were easily the most disabled, across all activities. Women with only lumbar pain were the least disabled. Interestingly, of the activities surveyed, shopping was much better tolerated than housework, exercise or walking for 20 min.

Management of low back pain should begin before onset[2], i.e. a careful history of back problems which may predispose to pain during pregnancy should be elicited, and if possible, addressed even before pregnancy. Education of the pregnant woman should include the possibility of back pain and the reasons why, leading to a program of daily low back and pelvic stretching and strengthening exercises. Proper posture and avoiding high-heeled shoes are good general recommendations. Strategies to help alleviate back pain once it has occurred include: elevating one foot on a low stool when standing or sitting; use of a low back cushion; changing position; analgesics; hot water baths or bottles; and stress management or relaxation techniques. Daily adherence to a low back stretching program will also help. Patients should be queried about specific disruptions which may respond better to particular treatments. Night-time pain may improve when the patient sleeps on her left side, relieving compression on the inferior vena cava. The rare patient with a lumbosacral radiculopathy may need bed-rest, traction, analgesia, custom-made lumbar corset[45], TENS (transcutaneous electrical stimulation) unit or even surgery, although the last should be avoided unless there is loss of bladder control or limb paralysis. The woman with symptoms of sacroiliac joint dysfunction may also benefit from rest, analgesia, acupuncture[46] or manipulation, and may need a trochanteric belt[13], a rigid cloth strapped around the pelvis to minimize movement in the sacroiliac joint and symphysis pubism (Figure 2). Electrodiagnostic testing and magnetic resonance imaging are probably best put off unless surgery is considered or neurologic deficits arise[41]. Pain during labor may respond to subcutaneous injections of sterile water over the sacrum and lower back[47,48], but apparently not to sterile saline[48]. The response is presumed to be related to the gate control theory of pain relief, similar to a TENS unit. Of course, epidural anesthesia is also useful in alleviating back pain during labor.

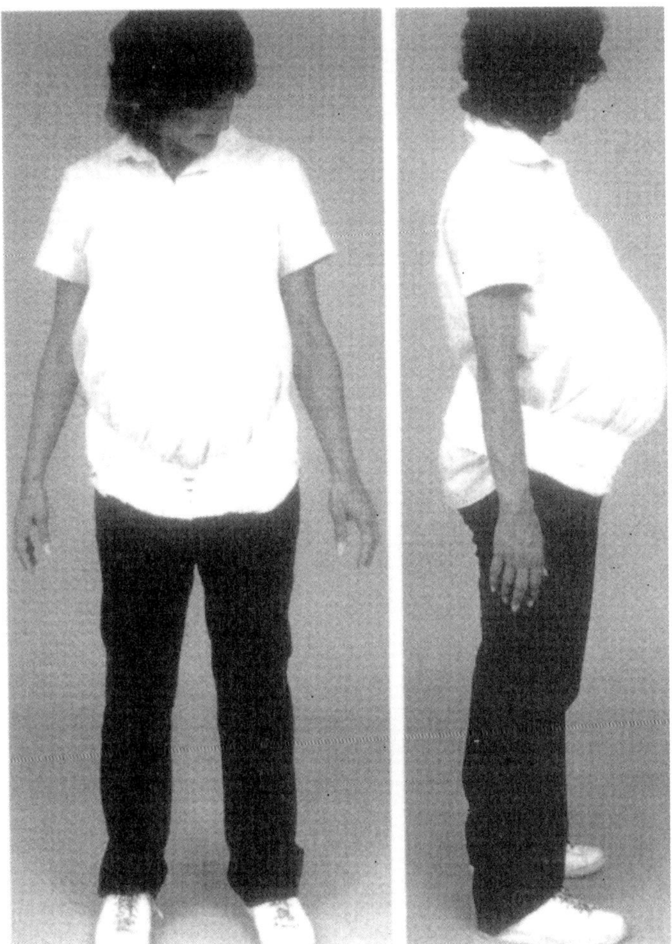

Figure 2 A properly worn trochanteric belt. Reproduced with permission from reference 13

References

1. Caillet R. *Low Back Pain Syndrome*. Philadelphia: FD Davis, 1987
2. Hainline B. Low-back pain. *Adv Neurol* 2002;90:9–23
3. Borenstein DG, Wiesel SW, Boden SD. *Low Back Pain. Medical Diagnosis and Comprehensive Management*, 2nd edn. Philadelphia: WB Saunders, 1995:10
4. Hummel P. *Changes in Posture during Pregnancy*. Philadelphia: WB Saunders, 1987
5. Abrahamson D, Roberts SM, Wilson PD. Relaxation of the pelvic joints in pregnancy. *Surg Gynecol Obstet* 1934;58:595–613
6. Young J. Relaxation of the pelvic joints in pregnancy. *J Obstet Gynaecol Br Emp* 1940;47:493–523

7. Zarrow M, Holmstron EG, Salhanick HA. The concentration of relaxin in the blood serum and other tissues of women during pregnancy. *J Clin Endocrinol* 1955;15:22–7
8. Cantin L. *Relâchement des symphysis et artralgies pelviennes d'origine gravidique*. Thesis, Paris, 1899
9. Calguneri M, Bird HA, Wright V. Changes in joint laxity occurring during pregnancy. *Ann Rheum Dis* 1982;41:126–8
10. Fast A, Weiss L, Parikh S, Hertz G. Night backache in pregnancy. *Am J Phys Med Rehab* 1989;68:227–9
11. Turgut F, Turgut M, Mentes E. Lumbosacral plexus compression by fetus: an unusual cause of radiculopathy during teenage pregnancy. *Eur J Obstet Gynecol Reprod Biol* 1997;73:203–4
12. Mantle MJ, Greenwood RM, Currey HLF. Backache in pregnancy. *Rheum Rehab* 1977;16:95–101
13. Heckman JD, Sassard R. Current concepts review: musculoskeletal considerations in pregnancy. *J Bone Joint Surg* 1994;11:1720–30
14. Fast A, Shapiro D, Ducommun EJ, *et al*. Low-back pain in pregnancy. *Spine* 1987;12:368–71
15. Berg G, Hammar M, Moller-Nielsen J, *et al*. Low back pain during pregnancy. *Obstet Gynecol* 1988;71:71–5
16. Orvieto R, Achiron A, Ben-Rafael Z, *et al*. Low-back pain in pregnancy. *Acta Obstet Gynecol Scand* 1994;73:209–14
17. Ostgaard HC, Roos-Hansson E, Zetherstrom G. Regression of back and posterior pelvic pain after pregnancy. *Spine* 1996;21:2777–80
18. Sturesson B, Uden G, Uden A. Pain pattern in pregnancy and 'catching' of the leg in pregnant women with posterior pelvic pain. *Spine* 1997;22:1880–3
19. Larsen EC, Wilkin-Jensen C, Hansen A, *et al*. Symptom-giving pelvic girdle relaxation in pregnancy. I: Prevalence and risk factors. *Acta Obstet Gynecol Scand* 1999;78:105–10
20. Albert H, Godskesen M, Westergaard J. Evaluation of clinical tests used in classification procedures in pregnancy-related pelvic joint pain. *Eur J Spine* 2000;9:161–6
21. Noren L, Ostgaard S, Johansson G, *et al*. Lumbar back and posterior pelvic pain during pregnancy: a 3-year follow-up. *Eur Spine J* 2002;11:267–71
22. Albert HB, Godskesen M, Westergaard JG. Incidence of four syndromes of pregnancy-related pelvic joint pain. *Spine* 2002;27:2831–4
23. Nilsson-Wikmar L, Harms-Ringdahl K, Pilo C. Back pain in women postpartum is not a unitary concept. *Physiother Res Int* 1999;4:201–13
24. Kristiansson P, Svardsudd K, von Schoultz B. Serum relaxin, symphyseal pain, and back pain during pregnancy. *Am J Obstet Gynecol* 1996;175:1342–7
25. Reginald PW, Beard RW, Kooner JS, *et al*. Intravenous dihydroergotamine to relieve pelvic congestion with pain in young women. *Lancet* 1987;1:351–3
26. Melzack R, Schaffelberg D. Low-back pain during labor. *Am J Obstet Gynecol* 1987;156:901–5
27. Laslett M, Williams M. The reliability of selected pain provocation tests for sacroiliac joint pathology. *Spine* 1994;19:1243–9
28. McCombe PF, Fairbank JCT, Cockersole BC, *et al*. Reproducibility of physical signs in low back pain. *Spine* 1989;14:908–18

29. Potter NA, Rothstein JM. Intertester reliability for selected tests of the sacroiliac joint. *Phys Ther* 1985;65:1671–5
30. Mens JMA, Vleeming A, Snijders CJ, *et al.* Responsiveness of outcome measurements in rehabilitation of patients with posterior pelvic pain since pregnancy. *Spine* 2002;27:1110–15
31. Ostgaard HC, Zetherstrom G, Roos-Hansson E. The posterior pelvic pain provocation test in pregnant women. *Eur Spine J* 1994;3:258–60
32. Vleeming A, de Vries HJ, Mens JMA, *et al.* Possible role of the long dorsal sacroiliac ligament in women with peripartum pelvic pain. *Acta Obstet Gynecol Scand* 2002;81:430–6
33. Mens JMA, Vleeming A, Snijders CJ, *et al.* Validity of the active straight leg raise test for measuring severity in patients with posterior pelvic pain after pregnancy. *Spine* 2002;27:196–200
34. Padua L, Padua R, Bondi R, *et al.* Patient-oriented assessment of back pain in pregnancy. *Eur Spine J* 2002;11:272–5
35. Brynhildsen J, Hansen A, Persson A, *et al.* Follow-up of patients with low back pain during pregnancy. *Obstet Gynecol* 1998;91:182–6
36. Ostgaard HC. Assessment and treatment of low back pain in working pregnant women. *Semin Perinatol* 1996;20:61–9
37. LaBan MM, Perrin JCS, Latimer FR. Pregnancy and the herniated lumbar disc. *Arch Phys Med Rehab* 1983;64:319–21
38. LaBan MM, Viola S, Williams DA, *et al.* Magnetic resonance imaging of the lumbar herniated disc in pregnancy. *Am J Phys Med Rehab* 1995;74:59–61
39. Weinreb JC, Wolbarsht LB, Cohen JM, *et al.* Prevalence of lumbosacral intervertebral disk abnormalities on MR images in pregnant and asymptomatic nonpregnant women. *Radiology* 1989;170:125–8
40. Kelsey JL, Greenberg RA, Hardy RJ, *et al.* Pregnancy and the syndrome of herniated lumbar intervertebral disc; an epidemiological study. *Yale J Biol Med* 1975;48:361–8
41. Garmel SH, Guzelian GA, D'Alton JG, *et al.* Lumbar disk disease in pregnancy. *Obstet Gynecol* 1997;89:821–2
42. Egerman RS, Mabie WC, Eifrid M, *et al.* Sacroiliitis associated with pyelonephritis in pregnancy. *Obstet Gynecol* 1995;85:834–5
43. Macarthur AJ, Macarthur C, Weeks SK. Is epidural anesthesia in labor associated with chronic low back pain? A prospective cohort study. *Anesth Analg* 1997;85:1066–70
44. Ostgaard HC, Zethersrom G, Roos-Hansson E. Back pain in relation to pregnancy: a 6-year follow-up. *Spine* 1997;22:2945–50
45. Beaty CM, Bhaktaram VJ, Rayburn WF, *et al.* Low backache during pregnancy. Acute hemodynamic effects of a lumbar support. *J Reprod Med* 1999;44:1007–11
46. Wedenberg K, Moen B, Norling A. A prospective randomized study comparing acupuncture with physiotherapy for low-back and pelvic pain in pregnancy. *Acta Obstet Gynecol Scand* 2000;79:331–5
47. Labreque M, Nouwen A, Bergeron M, *et al.* A randomized controlled trial of nonpharmacologic approaches for relief of low back pain during labor. *J Fam Pract* 1999;48:259–63
48. Martensson L, Wallin G. Labour pain treated with cutaneous injections of sterile water: a randomized controlled trial. *Br J Obstet Gynaecol* 1999;106:633–7

5

Multiple sclerosis

P. K. Coyle and M. A. Hammad

OVERVIEW

After trauma, multiple sclerosis (MS) is the major acquired central nervous system (CNS) disorder of young adults. At least 400 000 Americans have MS, and up to two million people are affected worldwide. MS is organ-specific. Although the systemic immune system is up-regulated[1–3], and a limited number of reports suggest peripheral nervous system involvement[4–11], in fact the damage process appears to be confined to the brain and spinal cord.

Characteristics

This immune-mediated inflammatory demyelinating CNS disease shows characteristic features (Table 1). Most MS patients are women of child-bearing age[12,14]. The only exception is the primary progressive subtype, which shows an equal sex ratio and older age of onset[15,16]. Most MS patients are Caucasians (>90%) of Northern European, and especially Scandinavian, background. MS is rare among Asians, Africans, Latin-Americans and Native-Americans, with higher rates in African-Americans. Populations such as the Innuits and Hutterites in Canada, and the Lapps in Finland, show low rates of MS, despite being surrounded by populations with high rates. They appear to be resistant.

Clinical subtypes

MS shows a severity spectrum which ranges from an asymptomatic pathologic process (found on autopsy) to mild symptoms and to severe disabling disease[17]. Clinical presentation takes the form of relapsing disease (distinct attacks with clinical stability in between) or progression (slow worsening with accumulating neurologic deficits). Early in the disease, attacks commonly involve sensory, motor, cerebellar or visual problems. Later in the disease, bladder, bowel, sexual and cognitive

Table 1 Characteristic features of multiple sclerosis (MS)

Disease of young postpubertal adults
Very unusual (<1%) to have onset before age 10 or after age 60 years
90% of patients have onset between ages 15 and 50 years
Peak onset in early 20s
Average age at onset 28–30 (relapsing), 38–40 (progressive MS)
Female-predominant disease
70–75% of all patients are female[12–14]
Only primary progressive subtype shows equal sex ratio[13]
Caucasian disease
> 90% of cases
Mainly Northern European, Scandinavian background
Unusual in Asians, Africans, Latin-Americans, Native-Americans
Heterogeneous and variable disease
Disease may be asymptomatic or symptomatic (with relapsing or progressive course)
Disease course differs for every individual
There is genetic and immunologic heterogeneity
susceptibility genes differ based on racial group
acute lesions show several distinct patterns of immune damage

problems often develop. The first attack is more likely to be monoregional (involving a single system) than multiregional. Relapses develop over hours to days (rarely minutes to weeks), and by definition they must last for at least 24–48 h. The second attack occurs within a year in 30% of patients. When first-attack patients show multiple lesions on brain magnetic resonance imaging (MRI), over 80% will have another attack by year 10. The relapse rate is highest early in the disease, and falls over time. It is important to distinguish pseudoattacks (also called pseudoexacerbations) from genuine relapses. Pseudoattacks involve temporary neurologic deficits, which reflect disrupted nerve conduction through old, inactive lesions rather than *de novo* damage. They are most commonly seen with infection-related temperature and inflammatory metabolic changes, and deficits resolve as soon as the infection is controlled.

Four clinical subtypes are recognized, based on expert consensus (Table 2)[17]. No clear biologic markers distinguish these subtypes, and they are based strictly on observation of clinical disease pattern. It seems likely that patients who show slow worsening from the onset (primary progressive, progressive relapsing) form a close if not identical continuum. It is not clear whether all these progressive subtypes reflect the same pathologic process.

Table 2 Clinical subtypes of multiple sclerosis (MS)

Subclinical (asymptomatic)
May account for up to 20% of cases
Clinical (symptomatic)
Relapsing
85% of MS at onset, 55% of all cases
patients experience discrete disease attacks, with variable degrees of recovery
patterns remain clinically stable between attacks
Progressive
primary progressive
10% of MS
slow worsening from onset without relapses
older age of onset (on average 38–40 years)
equal sex ratio
progressive myelopathy (in 85%)
progressive relapsing
5% of MS
similar to primary progressive, except for later superimposed relapses
secondary progressive
30% of all MS
relapsing patient who transitions after a period of time to progressive disease; relapses become less common, and ultimately cease

Natural history

The typical MS patient starts out with relapses, but ultimately develops progressive disease. Life span is almost normal, shortened by just a few years[18]. In patients with significant disability, death may occur secondary to complications such as sepsis, aspiration pneumonia or decubiti. Rarely, MS can be a primary cause of death, owing to acute lesions in the low brainstem that affect vital cardiovascular and respiratory centers. Death can also occur from suicide, which is more common in the MS population as a result of the high rate of depression[19]. Although mortality is not an issue in MS, morbidity is a major one. Ultimately most patients become disabled, are unable to work and have limited mobility, requiring assistive devices.

Pathogenesis

MS involves genetic, environmental and immunologic factors. The disease appears to be heterogeneous, with patient subsets that may have somewhat distinct etiologies.

Table 3 The role of genetics in multiple sclerosis

Increasing identification of multiple involved genes susceptibility, protection and disease severity genes
Approximately 20% of patients report another affected relative some families show multiple affected members
Disease frequency (in the typical Caucasian population) is 0.2%; this increases to 3–5% with an affected first-degree relative[20]
Monozygotic twins show concordance rate of at least 25% vs. dizygotic twins (5%)[21] risk higher for female (34%) monozygotic twins vs. males (5%)

Although MS is not inherited (multiple searches of the human genome have failed to detect a critical gene), genetics clearly plays an important role in development and expression of the disease (Table 3).

Multiple environmental factors have been postulated to be important in the development of MS, but exposure to common pathogens is believed to be key (Table 4). Although it is possible that a subset of MS involves persistent CNS infection, the data best support that exposure to common viruses and bacteria in early childhood, in a way that is not yet understood, sets the stage for MS.

Molecular mimicry (shared epitope sequences or molecular configurations between pathogens and autoantigens, including CNS antigens) is well documented. It may be that infection-triggered cross-reactivity to a myelin or other CNS component initiates MS in genetically vulnerable individuals. Epitope spread occurs when CNS damage releases multiple sequestered antigens to the systemic immune system.

The host immune system is critical in the pathogenesis of MS (Table 5). Local immune reactions within the CNS result in tissue damage and the formation of plaques[24]. Plaques are small (in millimeters), but can coalesce into lesions a centimeter or more in size. They are characterized by early edema and inflammation, demyelination (myelin is stripped off by macrophages), axonal damage, gliosis, variable cell (oligodendrocyte, neuron) loss and remyelination (which is variable, and incomplete).

MS involves inflammation and neurodegeneration. The active ongoing damage process is markedly underestimated clinically. Axon and neuron involvement, which has only been highlighted in the past few years, may be as important as myelin and oligodendrocyte involvement.

Diagnosis

MS is misdiagnosed in about 5–10% of patients. This reflects, in large part, overinterpretation of an abnormal brain MRI. Diagnosis can also

Table 4 Environmental factors involved in multiple sclerosis (MS)

Geographic low-, medium-, and high-risk zones
little MS at the equator; cases increase as one moves north and south
Migration studies indicate risk of MS determined in childhood, the first 15 years of life
Reports of multiple small clusters, one major epidemic
Faeroe Isles: cases occurred within 3 years of exposure to British troops present from 1942 to 1945; there were three subsequent waves of MS cases[22]
Case numbers appear to be increasing in developed countries and among unusual nationalities
MS is on the rise as natural infections in early childhood are decreasing (through vaccination, improved sanitation, hygiene programs)
MS is becoming more common in China, India and the Middle East (areas and populations where the disease was previously rare)
MS is more common in patients with older age-onset childhood infections
Ubiquitous pathogens have been linked to subsets of MS
herpes agents: prior infection with Epstein–Barr virus (EBV) appears to be close to an absolute requirement for development of MS; some groups report active human herpes virus type 6 (HHV-6), B variant, in subsets of MS
retroviruses: some groups report an endogenous retrovirus in subsets of MS; both human immunodeficiency virus (HIV) and human T-cell lymphotrophic virus type 1 (HTLV-1) can produce neurologic syndromes which mimic MS
Chlamydia pneumoniae: some groups report active central nervous system (CNS) infection with this bacterial agent in a large proportion of MS
spirochetal infections (including *Borrelia burgdorferi*, the etiologic agent of Lyme disease): some groups report a subset of patients who have histopathologic evidence of spirochetes in brain tissue and cerebrospinal fluid (CSF) sediment
Infections can trigger MS relapses
data are strongest for ubiquitous viral pathogens including respiratory tract agents; data are accumulating for bacterial infections such as urinary tract infections

be delayed, particularly in women who present with transient neurologic symptoms that are attributed to stress. Appropriate diagnosis is important for therapy, for informed planning, to remove uncertainty and to improve sense of well-being.

MRI is the best current laboratory marker of disease activity in relapsing and secondary progressive MS. Typical abnormalities are scattered white matter lesions, which are hyperintense on T2 and proton density scans. Some 30–40% of these lesions will be hypointense on T1 scans, a sign of more severe tissue damage.

Table 5 Immunological factors in multiple sclerosis (MS)

The host immune system attacks the central nervous system (CNS)
- activated blood lymphocytes penetrate into the CNS and become involved in local immune responses
- there is local CNS cell (microglia, endothelium, astrocyte) activation and immune molecule up-regulation
- the resultant tissue damage produces MS plaques (the neuropathologic lesion of MS)
- CNS plaques form in preferential areas around venules and close to cerebrospinal fluid (CSF); they occur in waves, throughout the duration of MS
- most plaques (as judged by magnetic resonance imaging (MRI), 80–90%) are clinically silent and associated with a clinical relapse

Acute plaques show immunologic heterogeneity (four patterns)[23]
- macrophage-associated demyelination, with active remyelination and normal oligodendrocyte numbers (16%)
- antibody- and complement-mediated demyelination, with active remyelination and normal oligodendrocyte numbers (59%)
- distal dying-back oligodendrogliopathies without remyelination, and markedly reduced oligodendrocyte numbers, some lost by apoptosis (consistent with ischemic toxic or infectious oligodendrocyte injury) (24%)
- primary oligodendrocyte injury without remyelination and markedly reduced oligodendrocyte numbers (suggestive of metabolic injury) (2%)

MS involves variable injury to myelin, axons, oligodendrocytes and neurons, with reactive astrocytosis

Immune/inflammatory injury mechanisms include lymphocytes (T, B and natural killer cells), antibody/complement, cytokines/chemokines, nitric oxide/peroxynitrite, excitatory amino acids, matrix metalloproteinases

Cerebrospinal fluid (CSF) analysis provides complementary information to neuroimaging. It is particularly helpful in patients with atypical clinical syndromes, or normal or atypical brain MRI, or to establish a diagnosis of primary progressive MS. The most useful CSF test is detection of oligoclonal bands, followed by elevated immunoglobulin G (IgG) index (intrathecal IgG production). CSF cell counts of over 50 white blood cells/mm^3, and protein values over 100 mg/dl, suggest an alternative diagnosis.

Evoked potentials can provide evidence of subclinical lesions. Based on recent practice guidelines, they have a limited role in the diagnosis of

Table 6 International Panel (IP) McDonald criteria for magnetic resonance imaging (MRI)-based dissemination in space and time[26]

MRI dissemination in space
Three of four criteria:
- 1 Gd+ lesion, or 9 T2W hyperintense lesions
- ≥ 1 infratentorial lesion
- ≥ 1 juxtacortical lesion
- ≥ 3 periventricular lesions
  - lesions ordinarily > 3 mm
  - spinal cord lesion may substitute for brain lesion

MRI dissemination in time
- (A) First scan ≥ 3 months after clinical event
  - (1) Gd+ lesion (at independent site) demonstrates dissemination in time
  - (2) Gd– scan: follow up MRI ≥ 3 months; new T2 or Gd+ lesion demonstrates dissemination in time
- (B) First scan < 3 months after clinical event; on 2nd scan ≥ 3 months after event
  - (1) Gd+ lesion demonstrates dissemination in time
  - (2) Gd– scan: follow-up 3rd MRI ≥ 3 months after 1st; new T2 or Gd+ lesion disseminated in time

MS, with the exception of visual evoked potentials (VEPs)[25]. Selected blood tests are helpful to exclude alternative diagnoses or codiagnoses, including genetic disorders, infections, vitamin deficiencies, connective tissue diseases, antiphospholipid syndrome, paraneoplastic syndromes, endocrine disturbances, acanthocytosis and myasthenia gravis.

Formal criteria for the diagnosis of MS have been revised recently to include MRI. The International Panel (IP) McDonald criteria define MRI evidence for dissemination in space and time (Table 6)[26]. They also specify new criteria for the diagnosis of primary progressive MS (Table 7). The IP criteria specify diagnostic categories of MS, possible MS and not MS. They utilize MRI, CSF analysis and VEPs as adjunctive laboratory tests. The new diagnostic criteria provide a framework for documenting dissemination in time and space by clinical or MRI criteria (Table 8).

Treatment issues

The single most important advance in MS has been the development of disease-modifying therapies (DMTs), drugs which decrease damage from the disease. They include four immunomodulators and one immunosuppressive agent (Table 9).

The typical MS patient is a young woman of child-bearing age. There are important treatment issues for the patient who is pregnant,

Table 7 International Panel (IP) McDonald criteria for diagnosis of primary progressive multiple sclerosis[26]

(1) Abnormal CSF (positive oligoclonal bands, or elevated IgG index)

(2) Any one of the following:
- (a) ≥9 T2W brain MRI lesions
- (b) ≥2 spinal cord lesions
- (c) 4–8 brain + 1 cord lesion(s)
- (d) 4–8 brain lesions + abnormal VEP
- (e) < 4 brain + 1 cord lesion + abnormal VEP

(3) Dissemination in time by MRI, or continued progression for 1 year

CSF, cerebrospinal fluid; MRI, magnetic resonance imaging; VEP, visual evoked potential

Table 8 International Panel (IP) McDonald diagnostic criteria for relapsing multiple sclerosis

Clinical presentation	*Dissemination in space*	*Dissemination in time*
≥2 attacks; objective clinical evidence of ≥2 lesions	not needed	not needed
≥2 attacks; objective clinical evidence of 1 lesion	MRI criteria, or ≥2 MRI lesions + abnormal CSF, or new attack at new site	not needed
1 attack; objective clinical evidence of ≥2 lesions	not needed	MRI criteria, or 2nd attack
1 attack; objective clinical evidence of 1 lesion (CIS)	MRI criteria, or ≥2 MRI lesions + abnormal CSF	MRI criteria, or 2nd attack

CIS, clinically isolated syndrome; MRI, magnetic resonance imaging; CSF, cerebrospinal fluid

attempting to become pregnant or breast-feeding. In addition, MS involves a variety of symptomatic treatment issues. Glucocorticoids are routinely used to treat acute relapses. They appear to improve the time frame to recovery, and recent studies suggest they even improve the degree of recovery and lessen permanent tissue damage[27]. MS is associated with a series of symptoms including fatigue, cognitive deficits, depression, spasticity, tremor, bladder and bowel dysfunction, sexual problems and ambulation difficulties. These are often managed by drug

Table 9 Multiple sclerosis disease-modifying therapies

Class	*Agent*	*Recommended dose*	*FDA pregnancy category*	*Issues*
Immunomodulator: anti-inflammatory cytokine	Avonex® (IFN-β1a) Rebif® (IFN-β1a) Betaseron® (IFN-β1b)	30 μg IM once weekly 44 μg SC three times weekly 250 μg (8 million IU) SC every other day	C	abortofacients in animal models
Immunomodulator: random polymers of 4AA (T cell manipulator)	Copaxone® (glatiramer acetate)	20 mg SC once daily	B	no identified animal/human risk
Broad spectrum immunosuppressant	Novantrone® (mitoxantrone)	12 mg/m^2 IV every 3 months (to a lifetime maximum dose of 140 mg/m^2)	D	cell-toxic immuno-suppressive

4AA, amino acids; IFN, interferon; IM, intramuscular; SC, subcutaneous; IV, intravenous; FDA, Food and Drug Administration

treatments which have sex-mediated actions and implications for fertility. These issues are discussed in greater detail below.

Impact of multiple sclerosis on pregnancy

The available data are very reassuring that MS has no direct effect on pregnancy. The disease does not influence fertility, conception, fetal viability or delivery. There are no increases in ectopic pregnancies, spontaneous abortions, stillbirths or congenital malformations[28,29]. It is important that young women with MS are aware of this information.

Impact of pregnancy on multiple sclerosis

Until 1950 or so, pregnancy was discouraged in MS patients because it was considered to have a negative effect. Over the next few years several studies were published which failed to confirm this widely held impression[30–32].

Table 10 Immunosuppressive factors involved in pregnancy

Increasing hormone levels (estriol, progesterone, prolactin, glucocorticoids)
Shift from Th1 to Th2 cells, with ↓ cell-mediated immunity and ↑ humoral immunity; includes IC formation and production of blocking antibodies
Pregnancy-related immunoregulatory proteins α-fetoprotein and others
Cytokine changes (↑ IFN-τ, a ruminant pregnancy cytokine; ↑ IL-10; inhibition of IFN-γ by plasma factor)
Maternal/ fetal MHC class II disparity (no class II expression by trophoblast layer, suppression of antipaternal MHC-specific T cells)
Other suppressive factors late-pregnancy serum factor which suppresses T-cell activation in the EAE animal model of MS

Th, T helper; IC, immune complex; IFN, interferon; IL, interleukin; MHC, major histocompatibility complex; EAE, experimental allergic/autoimmune encephalomyelitis; MS, multiple sclerosis

Pregnancy is an immunosuppressive state, which has a potent effect on MS disease activity[33]. Relapses decrease in pregnancy, particularly during the third trimester. This probably reflects a combination of maternal, fetal and placental factors (Table 10). The pregnancy-associated decrease in clinical disease activity is supported by the limited available MRI data. In a study of two patients, pregnancy was associated with a dramatic decrease in active lesions. In one woman, no new lesions were noted from the second trimester onwards, while the other woman showed no lesions in the third trimester[34]. In both patients, MRI activity returned to prepregnacy levels by 1 month postpartum. The findings from this neuroimaging study are consistent with the European study on pregnancy-related relapses in MS (PRIMS study). The PRIMS study involved 254 women and 269 pregnancies. Most of the women (246) had relapsing MS. During the last trimester they showed a decreased relapse rate, 70% lower than that in the prepregnancy period. However, the attack rate rose to 70% above the prepregnancy level in the 3 months postpartum, before returning to baseline[35].

A subsequent report provided a 2-year follow-up of the PRIMS cohort. From postpartum month 4, the relapse rate remained at the prepregnancy level. Disability and relapse rate at 2 years were not affected by pregnancy, type of delivery, use of epidural anesthesia or breast-feeding[36].

Consistent with fewer relapses, data suggest that MS is less likely to present during pregnancy. In a retrospective study, the rate of onset of MS during the 9 months of pregnancy was half that in the 6 months postpartum[37]. In a population-based study of 100 patients, none had disease onset during pregnancy, while nine presented in the 8 months postpartum[38]. This study also noted an increased risk of MS in nulliparous compared with parous women, with the risk ratio for MS increasing with age.

Pregnancy does not seem to increase disability[39]. In fact, there are suggestive data that pregnancy may improve disease course and slow time to disability end-points[38,40,41]. However, anecdotal data suggest that progressive patients who become pregnant may not do as well as relapsing patients.

DISEASE-MODIFYING THERAPIES AND PREGNANCY

The recently revised National Multiple Sclerosis Society disease management consensus statement emphasizes that the current DMTs are not approved for use in women who are pregnant, attempting to become pregnant or breast-feeding[42]. These drugs have distinct pregnancy category ratings (Table 9). In certain animal models, interferon-β (IFN-β) has abortofacient activity.

The available data on pregnancy outcome in patients exposed to the DMTs has not suggested teratogenicity concerns. One pregnancy registry for subcutaneous IFN-β1a (Rebif®) involved 1400 women and 37 pregnancies. Cases were collected from clinical trials data (both placebo-controlled and extension studies), which had examined a range of IFN-β doses from 22 µg once a week to 44 µg three times a week. Of the 30 pregnant women who were on the drug or close to taking the drug, there were 13 (45%) healthy live births, two (6.9%) premature births, six (21%) elective abortions and eight (27.6%) spontaneous abortions, including one fetal death. One pregnancy was lost to follow-up[43].

Glatiramer acetate (Copaxone®) has the most extensive reported pregnancy registry, involving clinical trials and postmarketing surveillance. In 21 global clinical trials (placebo-controlled and open-label) involving 2380 women, there were 40 reported pregnancies[44]. For the 30 women whose pregnancy outcome was known (ten were lost to follow-up), there were 18 (60%) elective abortions, five (16.7%) spontaneous abortions, six (20%) healthy live births and one (3.3%) cleft lip anomaly. This last mother had used carbamazepine during pregnancy, and it was felt that the anomaly was most likely due to the anticonvulsant. The postmarketing surveillance involved 345 reported pregnancies. Most women discontinued the drug once they found out that they were pregnant. Over 90% had DMT exposure during their first trimester. One hundred and thirty women were either lost to follow-up, or did not have outcome data because they had not reached their due date. Of the 215 known outcomes, there were 155 healthy live births, 43 spontaneous abortions, nine elective abortions, one ectopic pregnancy, one still-birth and six congenital anomalies (failure to thrive, finger anomaly, cardiomyopathy, urethrostenosis, anencephaly, adrenal cyst). Overall, of the 245 pregnancies reported from clinical trials or postmarketing surveillance, 66% involved healthy live births, 20% spontaneous abortions, 11% elective abortions, 2.9% congenital anomalies, 0.4% ectopic pregnancies and 0.4% stillbirths.

Based on data from these registries, the immunomodulators (and particularly glatiramer acetate) do not appear to have significant adverse effects during pregnancy. In light of the Food and Drug Administration (FDA) and consensus guidelines, however, most neurologists do not use these drugs in pregnant patients. For MS patients on immunomodulators who wish to become pregnant, the most common practice is to discontinue the drug a month prior to attempting pregnancy.

STEROIDS AND PREGNANCY

Synthetic glucocorticoids (such as methylprednisolone, prednisone, dexamethasone) are used as symptomatic treatments to accelerate recovery from MS relapses. Pregnancy is not an absolute contraindication to their use. Glucocorticoids can be used in the second and third trimesters, but are generally avoided in the first trimester (a critical time for organogenesis). Clinical attacks that occur during pregnancy are treated with steroid protocols identical to those used in non-pregnant patients.

Glucocorticoids are excreted in breast milk, and can affect infant growth. They can also affect bone density by decreasing body calcium via inhibition of calcium reabsorption, increased calcium excretion and potentially secondary hyperparathyroidism. Sustained and intense treatment may lead to osteonecrosis such as aseptic necrosis of the femoral head, while chronic treatment may lead to osteoporosis with bone collapse and fracture. These negative consequences on bone can be minimized by proactive measures such as calcium and vitamin D supplements, physical activity, bone density monitoring and appropriate specific osteoporosis therapies.

DELIVERY AND ANESTHESIA

Mode of delivery has no effect on the disease course of MS[45]. Of the various types of anesthesia, only spinal anesthesia is not recommended.

Anecdotally it has been associated with increased relapses. Two spinal anesthesia studies suggested an association with an increased postpartum relapse rate[46,47]; a retrospective study suggested that a high concentration of bupivacaine (> 0.25%) was associated with relapses[48]. Although these are limited data, they have led to the suggestion that spinal anesthesia should be avoided in MS. In the PRIMS study, epidural anesthesia clearly had no effect on relapse rate[36].

POSTPARTUM THERAPY

Some 30–40% of postpartum women will experience clinical attacks. Prophylactic therapy with intravenous immunoglobulin (IVIG) has been used for this high rise period. In one study, nine MS patients with 12 previous childbirth-associated relapses were treated with 0.4 g/kg over 5 days shortly after giving birth, followed by IVIG at weeks 6 and 12. None went on to have clinical relapses[49]. In another study, 50 pregnant women with relapsing MS received either 60 g or 10 g of IVIG load within 24 h of delivery, followed by 10 g monthly for 6 months. The postpartum relapse rate in these treated women was 66% less than that predicted from the PRIMS study[50]. An ongoing study in Europe is looking at pulse IVIG in the postpartum period in a larger number of patients.

Provided that the patient does not breast-feed, it is logical to resume immunomodulator therapy as soon as possible after delivery although it lacks definitive data. Some clinicians are electing to treat with a combination strategy of the primary immunomodulator, along with pulse IVIG for 6 months.

BREAST-FEEDING

There are conflicting data regarding the impact of breast-feeding on MS. Two studies found that breast-feeding had no effect on MS, while a third study suggested a benefit[35,51,52]. In one retrospective study of 483 women with MS, the postpartum relapse rate was independent of breast-feeding status[52]. Although the initial PRIMS study suggested a protective effect of breast-feeding, the 2-year follow-up data did not find any effect on breast-feeding[36].

There are no good data available on whether the DMTs enter breast milk. In a single case report, a young lactating woman with malignant melanoma was treated with IFN-α at 30 million IU. Levels of IFN in breast milk were only minimally elevated compared with control milk (1551 IU/ml vs. 1249 IU/ml), suggesting that this IFN did not penetrate into breast milk in any significant quantity[53].

Based on FDA and consensus guidelines, DMTs are not be used in patients who elect to breast-feed.

GENETIC/REPRODUCTIVE COUNSELING

MS patients who wish to become pregnant can be advised that there is no negative effect of pregnancy on their disease in the short or long term. In fact, pregnancy may have a positive effect on prognosis. With regard to genetic counseling, there is a small but finite increased risk for MS in their child. All patients should be aware of the increased risk of relapse in the postpartum months. The extent of physical disability in the individual patient is a legitimate consideration in planning pregnancy. Necessary help can be arranged ahead of time in case of a postpartum relapse, and to allow the new mother to get extra rest.

When one parent has MS, risk for the child ranges from 3 to 5% vs. 0.2% in the general population. When both patients have MS, the risk increases to 31%.

USE OF ORAL CONTRACEPTIVES

Oral contraceptives do not appear to increase the risk of developing MS, or to affect the overall disease course[54]. Use of oral contraceptives may be associated with fewer symptoms, and less disability. Some MS patients using birth-control pills have shown less disability[29]. It has been said that women with MS are less likely to experience menstrual worsening of their disease if they are taking oral contraceptives.

SUMMARY

Since the typical MS patient is a young woman of child-bearing age, pregnancy is a very important topic. There are very reliable data that MS has no significant effect on fertility, ability to conceive, fetal viability or delivery. Pregnancy has a profound effect on MS. Relapses decrease during pregnancy, only to increase temporarily in the postpartum months. This potent effect on disease activity is probably related to a combination of immunosuppressive factors that are turned on and then abruptly turned off. Ongoing studies are attempting to identify these important factors.

Although immunomodulators do not appear to have significant adverse effects during pregnancy, current consensus recommendations are that they are not used during pregnancy. In contrast, glucocorticoids can be used (in the second and third trimesters) to treat acute relapses. Pregnancy should be carefully discussed with patients, including effects on disease activity, genetic risks, impact on treatment modalities and optimal management of the high-risk postpartum period.

References

1. Wandinger KP, Sturzebecher CS, Bielekova B, *et al.* Complex immunomodulatory effects of interferon-β in multiple sclerosis include the upregulation of T helper 1-associated marker genes. *Ann Neurol* 2001; 50:349–57
2. Huang WX, Huang P, Hillert J. Systemic upregulation of CD40 and CD40 ligand mRNA expression in multiple sclerosis. *Mult Scler* 2000;6: 61–5
3. Huang W-X, Huang MP, Gomes MA, Hillert J. Apoptosis mediators fasL and TRAIL are upregulated in peripheral blood mononuclear cells in MS. *Neurology* 2000;55:928–34
4. Pollock M, Calder C, Allpress S. Peripheral nerve abnormality in multiple sclerosis. *Ann Neurol* 1977;2:41–8
5. Rubin M, Karpati G, Carpenter S. Combined central and peripheral myelinopathy. *Neurology* 1987;37:1287–90
6. Thomas PK, Walker RW, Rudge P, *et al.* Chronic demyelinating peripheral neuropathy associated with multifocal central nervous system demyelination. *Brain* 1987;110:53–76
7. Poser CM. Demyelinating polyradiculitis and multiple sclerosis. *Arch Neurol* 1982;39:67
8. Eisen A, Paty D, Hoirch M. Altered supernormality in multiple sclerosis peripheral nerve. *Muscle Nerve* 1982;5:411–14
9. Bhatti MT, Schmalfuss IM, Williams LS, Quisling RG. Peripheral third cranial nerve enhancement in multiple sclerosis. *AJNR Am J Neuroradiol* 2003;24:1390–5
10. Van der Meijs AH, Tan IL, Barkhof F. Incidence of enhancement of the trigeminal nerve on MRI in patients with multiple sclerosis. *Mult Scler* 2002;8:64–7
11. Di Trapani G, Carnevale A, Cioffi RP, Massaro AR, Profice P. Multiple sclerosis associated with peripheral demyelinating neuropathy. *Clin Neuropathol* 1996;15:135–8
12. Duquette P, Pleines J, Girard M, Charest L, Senecal-Quevillon M, Masse C. The increased susceptibility of women to multiple sclerosis. *Can J Neurol Sci* 1992;19:466–71
13. Jacobs LD, Wende KE, Brownscheidle CM, *et al.* A profile of multiple sclerosis: The New York State Multiple Sclerosis Consortium. *Mult Scler* 1999;5:369–76
14. Minden SL, Marder WD, Harrold LN, Dor A. *Multiple Sclerosis: A Statistical Portrait*. Cambridge, MA: ABT Associates, 1993
15. McDonnell GV, Hawkins SA. Primary progressive multiple sclerosis: a distinct syndrome? *Mult Scler* 1996;2:137–41
16. Thompson AJ, Polman CH, Miller DH, *et al.* Primary progressive multiple sclerosis. *Brain* 1997;120:1085–96
17. Lublin FD, Reingold SC. Defining the clinical course of multiple sclerosis: results of an international survey. National Multiple Sclerosis Society (USA) Advisory Committee on Clinical Trials of New Agents in Multiple Sclerosis. *Neurology* 1996;46:907–11

18. Weinshenker BG. Epidemiology of multiple sclerosis. *Neurol Clin* 1996; 14:291–308
19. Sadovnick AD, Eisen K, Ebers GC, Paty DW. Cause of death in patients attending multiple sclerosis clinics. *Neurology* 1991;41:1193–6
20. Robertson NP, Compston DAS. Prognosis in multiple sclerosis: genetic factors. In Siva A, Kesselring J, Thompson AJ, eds. *Frontiers in Multiple Sclerosis*. London: Martin Dunitz, 1999:51–61
21. Sadovnick AD, Ebers GC. Genetics of multiple sclerosis. *Neurol Clin* 1995; 13:99–118
22. Elian M, Dean G. Multiple sclerosis among the United Kingdom-born children of immigrants from the West Indies. *J Neurol Neurosurg Psychiatry* 1987;50:327–32
23. Lucchinetti C, Bruck W, Parisi J, Scheithauer B, Rodriguez M, Lassmann H. Heterogeneity of multiple sclerosis lesions: implications for the pathogenesis of demyelination. *Ann Neurol* 2000;47:707–17
24. Storch M, Lassmann H. Pathology and pathogenesis of demyelinating diseases. *Curr Opin Neurol* 1997;10:186–92
25. Gronseth GS, Ashman EJ. Practice parameter: the usefulness of evoked potentials in identifying clinically silent lesions in patients with suspected multiple sclerosis (an evidence-based review). *Neurology* 2000;54:1720–5
26. McDonald WI, Compston A, Edan G, *et al.* Recommended diagnostic criteria for multiple sclerosis: guidelines from the International Panel on the diagnosis of multiple sclerosis. *Ann Neurol* 2001;50:121–7
27. Zivadinov R, Rudick RA, De Masi R, *et al.* Effects of IV methylprednisolone on brain atrophy in relapsing–remitting MS. *Neurology* 2001;57; 1239–47
28. Sadovnick AD, Baird PA. Reproductive counseling for multiple sclerosis patients. *Am J Med Genet* 1985;20:349–54
29. Poser S, Raun NE, Wikstrom J, Poser W. Pregnancy, oral contraceptives and multiple sclerosis. *Acta Neurol Scand* 1979;59:108–18
30. Muller R. Studies on disseminated sclerosis. *Acta Med Scand* 1949;S222: 1–214
31. Tillman AJB. The effect of pregnancy on multiple sclerosis and its management. *Res Publ Ass Res Nerv Ment Dis* 1950;28:548–82
32. McAlpine D, Compston N. Some aspects of the natural history of disseminated sclerosis. *Q J Med* 1952;21:135–67
33. Abramsky O. Pregnancy and multiple sclerosis. *Ann Neurol* 1994;36: S38–41
34. Van Walderveen MA, Tas MW, Barkhof F, *et al.* Magnetic resonance evaluation of disease activity during pregnancy in multiple sclerosis. *Neurology* 1994;44:327–9
35. Confavreux C, Hutchinson M, Hours MM, *et al.* Rate of pregnancy-related relapses in multiple sclerosis. *N Engl J Med* 1998; 339:285–91
36. Confavreux C, Vukusic S, Adeleine P, *et al.* Pregnancy and multiple sclerosis (the PRIMS study): two-year results. *Neurology* 2001;56:A197
37. Poser S, Poser W. Multiple sclerosis and gestation. *Neurology* 1983;33: 1422–7

38. Runmarker B, Andersen O. Pregnancy is associated with a lower risk of onset and a better prognosis in multiple sclerosis. *Brain* 1995;118: 253–61
39. Lorenzi AR, Ford HL. Multiple sclerosis and pregnancy. *Postgrad Med J* 2002;78:460–4
40. Damek DM, Shuster EA. Pregnancy and multiple sclerosis. *Mayo Clin Proc* 1997;72:977–89
41. Verdru P, Theys P, Hooghe MB, Carton H. Pregnancy and multiple sclerosis: the influence on long term disability. *Clin Neurol Neurosurg* 1994; 96:38–41
42. NMSS Expert Opinion Paper. *Disease management consensus paper*, National Multiple Sclerosis Society, 2002, http://www.nationalmssociety.org/pdf/forpros/Exp_Consensus.pdf
43. Sandberg-Wollheim M for the Rebif Investigators. Outcome of pregnancy during treatment with interferon-β-1A (Rebif) in patients with multiple sclerosis. *Neurology* 2002;58:A455
44. Coyle PK, Johnson K, Pardo L, Stark Y. Pregnancy outcomes in patients with multiple sclerosis treated with glatiramer acetate (Copaxone®). *Neurology* 2003;60(Suppl 1):P01.11
45. Flachenecker P, Hartung HP. Multiple sclerosis and pregnancy. Overview and status of the European multicenter PRIMS study. *Nervenarzt* 1995;66:97–104
46. Stenuit J, Marchand P. Sequelae of spinal anesthesia. *Acta Neurol Psychiatry Belg* 1968;68:626–35
47. Bamford C, Sibley W, Laguna J. Anesthesia in multiple sclerosis. *Can J Neurol Sci* 1978;5:41–4
48. Bader AM, Hunt CO, Datta S, *et al*. Anesthesia for the obstetric patient with multiple sclerosis. *J Clin Anesth* 1988;1:21–4
49. Achiron A, Rotstein Z, Noy S, Mashiach S, Dulitzky M, Achiron R. Intravenous immunoglobulin treatment in the prevention of childbirth-associated acute exacerbations in multiple sclerosis: a pilot study. *J Neurol* 1996;243:25–8
50. Haas J. High dose IVIG in the postpartum period for prevention of exacerbations in MS. *Mult Scler* 2000;6(Suppl 2):S18–20; discussion S33
51. Pisacane A, Impagliazzo N, Russo M, Valiani R, *et al*. Breast feeding and multiple sclerosis. *Br Med J* 1994;308:1411–12
52. Nelson LM, Franklin GM, Jones MC, and the Multiple Sclerosis Study Group. Risk of multiple sclerosis exacerbation during pregnancy and breast-feeding. *J Am Med Assoc* 1988;259:3441–3
53. Kumar AR, Hale TW, Mock RE. Transfer of interferon α into human breast milk. *J Hum Lact* 2000;16:226–8
54. Villard-Mackintosh L, Vessey MP. Oral contraceptives and reproductive factors in multiple sclerosis incidence. *Contraception* 1993;47:161–8

6

Peripheral nerve disorders during pregnancy

J. M. Washington

INTRODUCTION

The management of peripheral nerve disorders during pregnancy can pose a unique challenge to neurologists and obstetricians. The opportunity to treat these disorders during pregnancy may arise for a number of reasons. The physiologic changes associated with pregnancy can predispose to peripheral nerve disorders. Patients with pre-existing peripheral nerve disease may become pregnant. The puerperium by nature may result in peripheral nerve injury. In each category of disease, management is complicated by the need to consider multiple variables when diagnostic and therapeutic decisions are made. The clinician is required to manage with the knowledge of the effect of pregnancy on the course of disease, and of the effect of disease and therapeutic choices on the pregnancy.

The disorders are grouped according to the time of presentation during pregnancy. Some of these disorders occur during multiple pregnancy stages. For example, facial neuropathy may present in the antenatal and postpartum periods. The peripheral nerve disorders that present during the antenatal period are primarily mononeuropathies. The management of peripheral nerve disorders that are not specific to pregnancy may be necessary during the antenatal period. Pregnancy dictates special considerations in the diagnosis and management of these disorders. The management of pre-existing disorders during the antenatal period may present specific therapeutic challenges. Peripheral nerve injuries at the time of delivery, the puerperium, are unique to pregnancy. The postpartum period is a common time for the recognition of peripheral nerve disorders. With the exception of facial neuropathy, the actual onset of disease is during the antenatal and puerperal periods.

The effective management of patients with peripheral nerve disorders during each stage of child-bearing frequently requires a combined effort from the treating neurologist and obstetrician. Communication and mutual understanding of basic pathophysiology and treatment modalities allow for improved patient outcome.

FOCAL PERIPHERAL NERVE DISORDERS DURING THE ANTENATAL PERIOD

Carpal tunnel syndrome

The incidence of carpal tunnel syndrome (Table 1) is increased during pregnancy. Carpal tunnel syndrome is reported to occur in 2–25% of pregnant women[1–4]. There is evidence to document that up to 62% of pregnant women have complaints of hand symptoms[3]. A small portion of these patients are referred for specialist and neurodiagnostic evaluation. For this reason, the true incidence of the disorder in pregnancy is probably higher.

The carpal tunnel is an anatomical compartment of the hand. The transverse carpal ligament is the superior border of the compartment. The inferior border consists of the carpal bones. The median nerve, flexor tendons and associated synovia are contained in the compartment. Median neuropathy at or distal to the wrist may result from edema or inflammation of the nerve or surrounding structures. Carpal tunnel syndrome associated with pregnancy has been attributed to a number of factors. These include redistribution of fluids, hormonal changes, tenosynovitis and pyridoxine deficiency[5]. The pathophysiology of the syndrome in pregnancy remains controversial. The actual mechanisms for its increased occurrence are probably multifactorial. Evidence, however, suggests that edema plays a more significant role during pregnancy. Carpal tunnel syndrome was twice as common in pregnant patients who had edematous hands when compared with those without edema of the hands[6]. Additional evidence

Table 1 Common nerve injuries in the antenatal period

Syndrome	*Nerve*
Carpal tunnel syndrome	median nerve
Meralgia paresthetica	lateral femoral cutaneous nerve
Iliohypogastric entrapment	iliohypogastric nerve
Bell's palsy	facial nerve
Parsonage–Turner	brachial plexopathy

of the increased role of edema is the increased incidence in older primiparous women with generalized edema[1].

Clinical features associated with an increased risk of development include older age, excessive weight gain, toxemia of pregnancy, edema and a history of carpal tunnel syndrome in previous pregnancies. In addition, the incidence of carpal tunnel syndrome was reported to triple in populations of women as smoking increased from zero to 25 or more cigarettes per day[7]. Smoking during pregnancy may lead to increased susceptibility to the disorder.

Carpal tunnel syndrome occurs most frequently during the third trimester of pregnancy, but may occur during the first and second trimesters. An incidence of 2% during the first trimester and 20% during the second trimester has been reported[4]. Postpartum onset of carpal tunnel syndrome has been reported in relatively older primiparous patients who breast-fed[4,8].

Paresthesias, loss of sensation and pain of the hand are typical clinical symptoms. The pain associated with the syndrome may at times extend to the forearm and upper arm. Physical examination may reveal the presence of Tinel's and/or Phalen's signs. Objective sensory loss and weakness are rare. The syndrome can frequently involve both upper extremities. The symptoms are exacerbated by repetitive use of the hands. Symptoms may occur exclusively or worsen at night. This phenomenon is related to the redistribution of fluid to dependent portions of the body during supine posture.

Asymptomatic median neuropathy during pregnancy has been documented with the use of nerve conduction studies[9]. The significance of this finding to future recurrence of carpal tunnel syndrome has yet to be determined. Neurodiagnostic measures were shown to parallel clinical improvement in one report[10]. The use of nerve conduction studies and electromyography is reserved for refractory cases, and in those patients with atypical weakness and pain. The clinical evaluation should include investigation for possible diabetes and hypothyroidism. These disorders are secondary causes for carpal tunnel syndrome, and also occur with increased frequency during pregnancy.

Carpal tunnel syndrome in non-pregnant patients is frequently treated with resection of the transverse carpal ligament when severe. The recommended approach to therapy for pregnancy-related carpal tunnel syndrome is conservative because the course is usually benign. Symptoms resolve spontaneously following delivery and with the use of wrist splints in most patients[11]. A prospective study of 40 patients reported that 82% of patients had good relief of symptoms after 2 weeks of night-time splint use[1]. Improvement of symptoms may be apparent as early as 1 week after splinting[11]. Local injection of corticosteroids is a second-line therapy. Hydrochlorthiazide has been recommended for patients with hand edema and symptoms[12]. Conservative measures are more likely to fail in patients with a prenatal history of carpal tunnel syndrome, onset during the first and second trimesters and a specific abnormality on physical examination. Poor response to conservative measures was documented in patients with both a positive Phalen's test within less than 30 s and abnormal two-point discrimination at the fingertips[4]. Carpal tunnel syndrome may result in permanent disability if left untreated. For this reason, patients with persistent symptoms should be evaluated with electrodiagnostic testing. In the case of axonal loss and loss of nerve potentials (as defined by electrodiagnostic testing), early surgical management should be considered.

Carpal tunnel syndrome with onset during pregnancy has a benign course in the majority of patients. Ekman-Ordeberg and colleagues reported complete relief of symptoms, 2 weeks postpartum, in 95% of patients[1]. The remaining 5% had resolution of symptoms 4 weeks after delivery. In severe cases the course of carpal tunnel syndrome may be associated with persistence of symptoms for more than 2 years after delivery[13]. Al Quattan and colleagues reported that patients with mild residual symptoms may initially respond to conservative therapy, but may require surgical release 2–16 years later[13]. Long-term follow-up of all patients with residual symptoms after delivery is recommended.

Meralgia paresthetica

Meralgia paresthetica is a syndrome produced by compression of the lateral femoral cutaneous nerve at the inguinal ligament. The lateral femoral cutaneous, a purely sensory nerve, exits the pelvis beneath the inguinal ligament. The symptom complex includes pain, paresthesias and loss of sensation of the anterior and lateral portion of the thigh. Symptoms can be bilateral in many cases[14]. The onset of symptoms is usually after week 30 of gestation. Diabetes and obesity are risk factors for development of the sensation during pregnancy. Decreased sensation to pain in the distribution of the nerve is the sole clinical finding. The nerve is purely sensory in function; thus, weakness of leg extension or thigh adduction suggests femoral neuropathy, obturator neuropathy or lumbar plexopathy. Objective evidence of nerve involvement and extent of injury may be documented with an abnormal nerve conduction study of the lateral femoral cutaneous nerve. This study may show a response of decreased amplitude or absence of the response.

Conservative therapy is recommended because pain and paresthesias typically resolve within 3 months of delivery[14]. Local injection of bupivocaine at the site of nerve entrapment may aid diagnosis and usually provides temporary symptomatic relief. Amitriptyline therapy may be useful in the treatment of residual postpartum symptoms.

Surgical decompression is rarely necessary for persistent refractory pain in the postpartum period.

Iliohypogastric neuropathy

Iliohypogastric nerve entrapment may occur during pregnancy, or rarely during the postpartum period[15]. The syndrome occurs spontaneously in 1/3000 to 1/5000 pregnancies[16]. The pain of the syndrome is severe, persistent and localized to the lower quadrant of the abdomen, flank or inguinal region. Increased sensitivity of the skin to touch in the area of pain is frequently associated. The entrapment occurs during pregnancy owing to the rapid expansion of the growing uterus. The growth of the uterus results in a stretch of the abdominal wall. This stretch results in tension on the iliohypogastric nerve as it exits the internal oblique, external oblique and transverse abdominus muscles. The diagnosis is based on clinical findings alone, and is dependent on documentation of sensory loss in the distribution of the nerve. Exclusion of other diagnostic considerations is imperative. The differential diagnosis includes appendicitis, renal colic, urinary tract infection, abruptio placentae and pyelonephritis.

The diagnosis can be confirmed by iliohypogastric nerve block. The condition is usually self-limited, but may require intervention when pain is intolerable. Injection of bupivocaine results in complete pain relief within minutes. Cryoneurolysis has been used to treat the condition in refractory cases[17].

Facial neuropathy

Charles Bell first described isolated facial nerve paralysis of acute onset in 1930. At the time of description, Bell also suggested an association with pregnancy and the postpartum period[18]. Subsequent reports have documented the incidence of idiopathic facial neuropathy or Bell's palsy in pregnancy.

The incidence of Bell's palsy in pregnancy is three times that in non-gravid women of child-bearing age[19]. The incidence has been reported to be 38–45.1/100 000 births[19,20], compared with 17/100 000 per year for non-pregnant women of child-bearing age. The incidence is yet greater in the third trimester and immediate postpartum period. Combined evidence from retrospective studies gives an incidence during these periods of 118 cases per 100 000 per year[19]. This indicates that the incidence during the third trimester and early postpartum period is six times that in non-pregnant women of child-bearing age[21]. The initial observation by Bell has been documented and has led to a number of hypotheses regarding the etiology of the neuropathy during pregnancy.

The explanation for this increased incidence of facial neuropathy during pregnancy is controversial. Most possible explanations are related to the changes in physiology that occur during pregnancy. A popular hypothesis relates to the immunosuppression of pregnancy and the herpes simplex virus. This immunosuppression is known to be at a peak during the last trimester of pregnancy. This state may result in reactivation of the herpes simplex virus. The immunosuppression may also result in an increased susceptibility to acquisition of the herpes virus[22]. Previous immunofluorescent and serological studies indicate that Bell's palsy is due to an immune reaction to the herpes virus[22]. Another hypothesis relates to vasa nervosum thrombosis due to the hypercoagulopathy of pregnancy. A relationship to increased total body and facial nerve water is reasonable[19,23]. An association between facial neuropathy and eclampsia (a state characterized by edema) has been reported[23,24]. The explanation for the phenomenon in pregnancy is probably multifactorial.

The evaluation of Bell's palsy in pregnancy includes an assessment of symptoms, physical findings and in some cases electrodiagnostic testing. The symptoms of facial neuropathy during pregnancy are similar to those in non-pregnant patients. Symptoms of pain in the cheek or ear, and ringing in the ears, typically occur suddenly. These symptoms may precede facial weakness. Facial weakness, however, usually develops within hours of these symptoms. Associated symptoms of hyperacusis, numbness of the face and/or tongue, drooling and eye dryness are common. Patients may also be aware of a loss of taste on the anterior two-thirds of the tongue. Clinical examination reveals unilateral muscle weakness of the brow, obicularis oculus and obicularis oris. Weakness of minor muscles of the face such as the platysma is present but may not be clinically apparent.

The clinical presentation must be distinguished from a supranuclear lesion that could be an indication of stroke. Supranuclear lesions of the facial nerve are distinguished by a sparing of the brow muscles on the affected side. Additional diagnostic considerations include trauma to the nerve owing to fracture of the petrous bone, middle ear and mastoid lesions and cerebellopontine angle tumors. Sarcoidosis and diabetes may also present with facial neuropathy. For this reason, systemic illness should be excluded.

Motor nerve conduction studies and blink reflex studies have been used to document the extent of injury for the purpose of prognostication. Normal facial nerve motor conduction studies 2–3 weeks after the onset of symptoms is associated with a complete recovery rate of 90%[25]. The addition of electrodiagnostic testing may supplement the management after the diagnosis is made by clinical history and examination.

Prognosis for recovery is excellent overall. Recovery of function is similar to that in the general population. Full recovery is expected in the majority of patients[24–26]. Spontaneous recovery without treatment is expected in 75% of patients with Bell's palsy. Previously, Bell's palsy in pregnancy was associated with a better prognosis than non-pregnancy-related neuropathy. In early retrospective studies a 90% recovery rate within 24 h to 80 days of onset was reported[20,23]. A more recent study reported a significantly lower recovery rate. The increased rate was related to the degree of nerve impairment. Prognosis for complete recovery was significantly worse for pregnant patients with complete facial paralysis. Gillman and associates reported a recovery rate of 52% in pregnant patients whose facial paralysis was complete 2 days after onset. This compared with a recovery rate of 77–88% in control patients. They also reported a recovery rate of 100% in all patients with incomplete paralysis[27]. This study clearly delineates differences in prognosis related to the severity of disease. These differences should be considered when treatment decisions are made.

Supportive therapy with the use of artificial tears and patching of the lid to prevent corneal abrasion is indicated in all patients. Surgical intervention may be considered if paralysis persists for 6–12 months. In the non-pregnant population, treatment with high-dose prednisone may accelerate recovery and reduce the incidence of aberrant regeneration[28]. Acyclovir has also been commonly used in the same group for therapy. Clinical experience has documented the safety of both agents during pregnancy. Treatment with either agent remains controversial during pregnancy. Treatment is thought to be superfluous by some because of the overall good prognosis in the majority of pregnant patients. Treatment with prednisone and acyclovir should be considered in pregnant patients with complete lesions because of more recent reports of poorer prognosis for complete recovery.

Plexopathy during pregnancy

Brachial plexopathy during pregnancy has been rarely reported[29–31]. Common symptoms of brachial plexopathy include pain, weakness, atrophy and sensory abnormalities of the shoulder girdle and upper extremity. Two citations reported patients with plexopathy and an underlying hereditary nerve disorder. One case was related to a presumed inflammatory neuropathy. Klein and colleagues demonstrated a significant inflammatory response in a small group of patients with related hereditary neuropathy with susceptibility to pressure palsy[29].

Lumbar plexopathy is included in the discussion of puerperal injuries below.

GENERALIZED PERIPHERAL NEUROPATHY IN THE ANTENATAL PERIOD

Acute inflammatory demyelinating polyradiculoneuropathy

Landry first described acute inflammatory demyelinating polyradiculoneuropathy in 1859. The description was later refined by Guillain, Barré and Strohl in 1916 and was subsequently named the Guillain–Barré syndrome[32]. The syndrome is currently called acute inflammatory demyelinating polyradiculoneuropathy or AIDP. The incidence of AIDP during pregnancy is 0.7–1.9/100 000 per year. This rate is comparable to the general population rate of 0.75–2 persons per 100 000 per year[33]. The classic syndrome of a subacute, progressive, paralyzing illness has been reported during pregnancy in more than 50 cases[34–38]. AIDP or Guillain–Barré syndrome during pregnancy poses a significant risk to the mother and fetus. Consideration of pregnancy-related issues in diagnosis and treatment results in a course and prognosis that is similar to that in the non-pregnant population, however.

The course of disease during pregnancy parallels the disease course in the general population[32]. The disorder is frequently a subacute, progressive, paralyzing illness. The syndrome presents with insidious onset of mild sensory and motor symptoms that may progress to ascending quadriparesis and respiratory function compromise within a matter of hours. An upper respiratory or gastrointestinal viral syndrome in some cases may precede the syndrome. Autonomic dysfunction is common in the syndrome. The diagnosis is apparent when ascending motor weakness is accompanied by areflexia and cerebrospinal fluid (CSF) cytoalbuminogenic disassociation. This mismatch of increased CSF protein levels and normal cells is also seen in chronic inflammatory demyelinating polyneuropathy (discussed below). Nerve conduction studies are used to document electrophysiologic evidence of demyelination in peripheral nerves.

The presentation during pregnancy poses special diagnostic considerations. Early symptoms may mimic those related to normal pregnancy. Symptoms of fatigue and non-specific numbness are common in pregnancy but may be the presenting symptoms of AIDP. Confusion regarding the etiology of these symptoms may result in delayed diagnosis and treatment. Delayed diagnosis could result in the onset of respiratory insufficiency outside a supportive environment. Treatment delays may lead to a worse prognosis. Treatment within the first 2 weeks of onset of symptoms is known to have an effect on prognosis for recovery of function[33]. The early diagnosis of antecedent infection is also most important during pregnancy. Identification of viral antecedent infections is important because of the clinical implications to mother and child. These implications may include mental retardation, microcephaly, congenital rubella, motor disorders, maternal fetal transmission of human immunodeficiency virus (HIV) and miscarriage. Cytomegalovirus, Epstein–Barr virus, varicella zoster virus, HIV and *Campylobacter jejuni* have been identified as infections that precede AIDP. Cytomegalovirus has been associated with 10–22% of AIDP cases[39,40]. Cytomegalovirus is a serious infection in the first trimester of pregnancy that leads to multiple early disabilities and later handicaps. Special consideration for the diagnosis of cytomegalovirus and other concurrent infection is advisable in all instances of AIDP during pregnancy.

The major effect of severe AIDP on pregnancy is a marked increase in the risk of premature birth[41,42]. This increased risk of premature birth may be related to maternal respiratory insufficiency and autonomic dysfunction.

The course of delivery in AIDP is not changed by the disease, but may be adversely altered by obstetric intervention[41]. Controlled studies of the effect of obstetric intervention on the course of AIDP have not been done, however. Induction of labor during the acute phase of illness may contribute to worsening of neurologic symptoms and is not recommended. Vaginal delivery at term is the preferred method of delivery. Assistance with the second stage of labor may be necessary owing to weakness of the abdominal muscles. Vaginal delivery assisted by prophylactic forceps or vacuum extraction has been recommended[41]. The strength of uterine contractions is not affected, owing to the smooth muscle architecture of the uterus. For this reason, AIDP is not a sole indication for the use of pitocin. Contractions of the uterus may be associated with autonomic hyper-reflexia. Cesarean section may be associated with deterioration of neurologic dysfunction[41]. The use of Cesarean section for delivery should be reserved for the patient who develops significant cardiac arrhythmia or severe hypertension. Decisions regarding obstetric intervention should include assessment of potential effects on the course of illness and progeny. These decisions should not be made on the sole basis of a diagnosis of AIDP.

Supportive care and careful monitoring of the patient's respiratory, cardiovascular and hemodynamic status are the mainstays of management[42]. The management of pregnant patients is similar to that of the general population. Periodic bedside monitoring of the patient's respiratory function and autonomic status and serial fetal assessment has been recommended. Vital capacity should be measured by spirometer several times a day. Intensive-care monitoring should be employed for patients with vital capacity measurements under 1.5 l, severe paresis and autonomic nervous system disturbances.

Therapeutic plasma exchange and intravenous immunoglobulin therapy are both effective in pregnant and non-pregnant patients. Therapeutic plasma exchange has a low risk of complication during pregnancy. Potential complications of this therapy include hypovolemia, volume overload and complications from catheter placement and maintenance. Experience with successful plasmapheresis during pregnancy has been documented[43]. There have been no prospective studies related to the safety of plasmapheresis in pregnancy. High-dose intravenous immunoglobulin has been shown to be at least as effective for therapy in AIDP in the non-pregnant population[44]. High-dose intravenous immunoglobulin has been safely used in autoimmune thrombocytopenia and immunodeficiency syndromes during pregnancy. The agent has also been used for the antiphospholipid syndrome and recurrent miscarriage without apparent adverse obstetric or maternal effect[45].

Chronic inflammatory demyelinating polyradiculoneuropathy

Peter Dyck and colleagues, in 1975, first described chronic inflammatory demyelinating polyneuropathy (CIDP)[46]. The syndrome is similar in pathophysiology and clinical presentation to acute demyelinating inflammatory polyneuropathy (AIDP). The clinical course and responses to therapy distinguish this syndrome from AIDP or Guillain–Barré syndrome. The syndrome of CIDP is characterized by symmetrical limb weakness, areflexia and sensory loss, with progression for at least 2 months' duration. In contrast to AIDP, respiratory insufficiency, facial weakness and autonomic dysfunction are relatively uncommon. These common complications of AIDP occur in less than 10% of cases of CIDP[47]. However, the effect of pregnancy on the course of the disease is not inconsequential. Since the original description in 1975, documentation of the clinical course of CIDP in pregnancy has been limited.

One series documented the course of CIDP in pregnancy and demonstrated an association of CIDP onset and relapse[48]. Among a series of 16 women of child-bearing age, the course of nine who became pregnant was reviewed. The onset of CIDP occurred during pregnancy in four of these patients. Relapse of pre-existing disease was reported in five of the patients. This series documented a worsening of symptoms during the third trimester and immediate postpartum periods. The study suggested an increased risk of relapse during pregnancy.

The diagnosis of CIDP is based on the clinical history of symptoms for at least 2 months, electrodiagnostic criteria, cytoalbuminogenic disassociation and rarely nerve biopsy. Electrodiagnostic criteria for definitive diagnosis must include at least four abnormalities on nerve conduction studies. These criteria include slowing of conduction velocity, prolongation of F-wave latency, prolonged distal motor latencies and conduction block in one or more nerves[49]. Examination of the CSF may or may not reveal an increase in protein without a coincident increase in cell count. Nerve biopsy examination may reveal evidence of inflammation and demyelination.

Treatment of CIDP during pregnancy is complicated by special considerations for maternal and fetal safety. The objective in therapy for CIDP is some form of immunomodulation, including corticosteroids, high-dose intravenous immunoglobulin, plasmapheresis and the use of various immunosuppressive therapies. The safe use of steroids during pregnancy and lactation has been documented[50]. The use of high-dose immunoglobulin and plasmapheresis is discussed above in relation to AIDP. Additional use of other immunomodulatory agents such as azathioprine and cyclophosphamide is common in the non-pregnant population. These agents should not be used during pregnancy and in patients of child-bearing age who wish to become pregnant. There is little documentation of issues of the puerperium in CIDP patients. The successful administration of spinal anesthetic has been reported[51].

Other generalized neuropathies during pregnancy

Few reports in the literature document the course of additional generalized polyneuropathies during pregnancy. One publication reported exacerbation of multifocal motor neuropathy (MMN) during the pregnancies of three patients[52]. MMN is classified as an inflammatory neuropathy like AIDP and CIDP. It differs from AIDP and CIDP in presentation, course and therapy. MMN is characterized by progressive asymmetric limb weakness without sensory deficits. Elevation of GM-1 antibody levels is frequently associated with the disorder. Nerve conduction studies document multifocal persistent conduction blocks of motor nerves with sparing of sensory nerves. Three cases of worsening of MMN during pregnancy were reported[52]. These patients experienced increased weakness, cramps, fasciculations and myokymic discharge during pregnancy. MMN is thought to be antibody-mediated, although a direct causal relationship of anti-GM-1 antibodies has not been established. All three patients were treated with high-dose intravenous immunoglobulin. The treatment resulted in improved strength and was not associated with complications. The authors postulated that the above exacerbations resulted from the suppression of humoral immunity that is present during pregnancy.

Severe postpartum axonal polyneuropathy was reported in two patients[53]. Both patients presented with acute weakness with nerve biopsy and electrodiagnostic studies consistent with axonal damage. The presentations did not meet diagnostic criteria for demyelinating neuropathy. Both were treated with plasmapheresis and had mild improvement. Motor weakness continued to improve over a period of months. These two cases may have represented the acute axonal sensory and motor variant form of acquired inflammatory neuropathies.

PERIPHERAL NERVE DISORDERS AT THE PUERPERIUM

Postpartum foot drop

Postpartum foot drop is the most common peripheral nerve disorder to occur at the puerperium (Table 2). The entity is most commonly a result of compression of the lumbosacral plexus by the fetal brow as it passes the brim of the pelvis[15]. The predominant involvement of the L4 and L5 segments of the lumbosacral trunk is manifested by weakness of the tibialis anterior, the major dorsiflexor of the foot. Pain and paresthesias of the lateral lower extremity may accompany weakness. The paralysis of foot dorsiflexion is unilateral when related to plexopathy. Lumbar plexopathy is more likely to occur in patients with short stature, large infants and primigravid state. Transverse rotation arrest during labor is an additional risk factor for postpartum foot drop[54].

Table 2 Puerperal nerve injuries

Injury	*Major manifestation*
Postpartum foot drop	
lumbar plexopathy	weakness of foot dorsiflexion
peroneal neuropathy	weakness of foot dorsiflexion
Femoral neuropathy	weakness of knee extension
Obturator neuropathy	weakness of thigh adduction
Pudendal neuropathy	urinary and fecal incontinence
Epidural anesthesia	
lumbar radiculopathy	lower-extremity weakness
spinal arachnoiditis	pain and weakness of the lower extremity
epidural hematoma	pain and weakness of the lower extremity
intraspinal injection	myelopathy
conus medullaris injury	lower-extremity weakness, urinary and fecal incontinence, lower-extremity pain and sensory loss

Foot drop diagnosed during the postpartum period has rarely been associated with distal peroneal neuropathy. Peroneal neuropathy has been related to prolonged squatting during natural childbirth[55]. Peroneal neuropathy as a result of the position of prolonged pressure by the hands while in knee hyperflexion has also been reported[56].

In my clinical experience, the prognosis for return of function has been excellent. The performance of nerve conduction studies and electromyography at least 2 weeks after delivery can document localization and aids in prognostic purposes. The latter can be reassuring to the patient and obstetrician.

Femoral neuropathy

Neuropathy of the femoral nerve during the puerperium was previously considered to be a rare occurrence. The incidence was reported by Vargo and colleagues in 1990 to be 2.8/100 000 cases[57]. The condition is probably more common than previously reported. Dar and associates reported an incidence of 1.5/1000 in a series of 400 deliveries in 1999[58]. An incidence of 1.1/100 was reported in an additional retrospective study[59]. The condition might be bilateral in some cases[60,61]. Risk factors for development include primiparity, prolonged labor and cephalopelvic disproportion. The entity is common and likely to be underreported.

The femoral nerve originates from the posterior divisions of the L2–L4 anterior rami. The nerve travels through the retroperitoneum between the psoas and iliacus muscles and then emerges from the pelvis under the inguinal ligament. The terminal portion of the nerve in the lower leg is the saphenous nerve. This nerve supplies sensory function to the medial speck of the lower extremity below the knee. Injury to the nerve may result in weakness of knee extension and hip flexion and impaired sensation of the anteromedial thigh. The physical examination is also remarkable for the absence of reflex at the knee on the involved side. Patients typically present during the first attempt to walk following delivery. The typical scenario includes collapse of one lower extremity at the knee as a result of quadriceps weakness. Weakness of lower-extremity extension may or may not be accompanied by paresthesias in the femoral sensory and saphenous nerve distributions.

The diagnosis of femoral neuropathy is based on the clinical history and examination findings noted in the above paragraph. Nerve conduction studies and electromyography are helpful in accurate localization of the injury and in determination of prognosis. Preservation of the femoral motor nerve and saphenous sensory response is associated with an excellent prognosis for recovery. These studies should be performed at least 2 weeks after injury. Electrodiagnostic studies may also aid the differentiation of intrapelvic from extrapelvic lesions. An intrapelvic localization may indicate the possibility of retroperitoneal hemorrhage or other space-occupying lesion. In the case of intrapelvic lesions, computed tomography or magnetic resonance imaging of the pelvis and retroperitoneum are indicated. An investigation for diabetes is also recommended because of increased frequency with this systemic illness.

The exact etiology for postpartum femoral neuropathy is not known. Possible mechanisms for nerve injury include compression of the nerve by a stretched inguinal ligament, pressure from the head of the fetus during labor, stretching of the nerve by excessive hip positioning in abduction and external rotation. The nerve may be more vulnerable to ischemic injury as a result of compression of the vasa nervorum. The neuropathy is not always associated with reasons for physical trauma. Postpartum femoral neuropathy has been reported following vaginal delivery and Cesarian delivery[62].

Management of postpartum femoral neuropathy should be conservative with reassurance. The prognosis for return of function is good. Improvement is expected within 2–8 weeks. The majority of patients will reach full recovery within 6 months[63].

Obturator neuropathy

Postpartum neuropathy due to compression of the obturator nerve has rarely been reported[64]. The neuropathy may be associated with postpartum femoral neuropathy. In isolation the syndrome of hypoesthesia of the medial thigh and weakness of thigh adductors is apparent. Prognosis for return of function is good.

Pudendal neuropathy

Pudendal nerve function may be compromised during vaginal delivery and may result in urinary and fecal incontinence and dysfunction. Electrodiagnostic studies of the pudendal nerve function before and after vaginal delivery were performed in 128 consecutive pregnant women[65]. In this group, a large fetus and prolonged second stage of labor correlated with significant prolongation of pudendal nerve distal latency. The study and others demonstrated that traumatic vaginal delivery might result in local damage to the pudendal nerves[65–67].

Pudendal nerve distal latency in electrodiagnostic studies has been used to document recovery in the nerve 2 months following vaginal delivery. Functional disturbance of pelvic floor muscles may persist for at least 6 months, however[67].

Complications of epidural anesthesia

The use of intrapartum epidural analgesia/anesthesia has increased over recent decades. The practice has been recognized to be a safe and effective method of pain relief during labor. The frequency of complications following epidural anesthesia is variable, and ranges from 0.01%[68–71]. Lumbar radiculopathy, polyradiculopathy and myelopathy secondary to conus medullaris injury[72] have been reported with spinal and combined spinal–epidural anesthesia. Lumbar epidural anesthesia was also reported as the etiology of a transient Horner's syndrome. The syndrome was postulated to be the result of inadvertent contact of the anesthesia with the thoracic spinal cord[73]. These complications may be associated with non-intentional administration of agents into the subarachnoid space during epidural procedures. As the use of epidural anesthesia becomes more common, the frequency of reported complications is likely to increase.

The mechanism of injury in most cases is uncertain. Mechanisms of injury that have been previously documented include direct injury to the nerve root by needle puncture, catheter insertion and intrafascicular injection[74]. Epidural hematomas might occur in the setting of prior coagulopathy. Epidural abscess might be seen in the setting of immunosuppression, bacteremia and prolonged catheterization. Spinal arachnoiditis may occur as a result of intrathecal injection of neurotoxic substances. These possible mechanisms should be considered in the immediate postpartum period.

Risk factors for anesthetic complications include lumbar stenosis, inadvertent subarachnoid administration of large volumes of highly concentrated preparations and longer duration of exposure to medications[74]. Intrathecal administration with unknown subarachnoid effects is discouraged. A prior predisposition to neuropathy may increase the susceptibility to anesthetic complications. A reported case of lumbar plexopathy in a patient with sickle cell anemia is one example[75].

The evaluation of suspected cases should include electromyography with nerve conduction studies and lumbar magnetic resonance imaging. Magnetic resonance imaging with gadolinium is recommended for two purposes. The first is to recognize potentially treatable causes for radiculopathy; these include epidural hematomas and pre-existing lumbar stenosis. The second purpose is the identification of lumbar arachnoiditis and intraspinal trauma as possible etiologies. The prognosis for return of function is largely dependent on the mechanism and extent of injury. In general, the prognosis has been good in the majority of patients.

References

1. Ekman-Ordeberg G, Salgeback S, Ordeberg G. Carpal tunnel syndrome in pregnancy. A prospective study. *Acta Obstet Gynecol Scand* 1987;66: 233–5
2. Gould JS, Wissinger HA. Carpal tunnel syndrome in pregnancy. *South Med J* 1978;71:144–5
3. McLennan HG, Oats N, Walstab J. Survey of hand symptoms in pregnancy. *Med J Aust* 1987;147:542–4
4. Stahl S, Blumenfeld Z, Yarnitsky D. Carpal tunnel syndrome in pregnancy: indications for early surgery. *J Neurol Sci* 1996;136:182–4
5. Atisook R, Benjapibal M, Sunsaneevithayakul P, Roongpisuthipong A. Carpal tunnel syndrome during pregnancy: prevalence of blood level of pyridoxine. *J Med Assoc Thai* 1995;78:410–14
6. Voitk AJ, Mueller JC, Farlinger DE, *et al.* Carpal tunnel syndrome in pregnancy. *Can Med Assoc J* 1983;128:277–81
7. Vessey MR, Villard-Mackintosh L, Yeates D. Epidemiology of carpal tunnel syndrome in women of child-bearing age. *Int J Epidemiol* 1990;19: 655–9
8. Wand JS. The natural history of carpal tunnel syndrome in lactation. *J R Soc Med* 1989;82:349–50
9. Snell NJ, Coysh HI, Snell BJ. Carpal tunnel syndrome presenting in the puerperium. *Practitioner* 1995;224:191–3
10. Weimer LH, Yin J, Lovelace RE, Gooch CL. Serial studies of carpal tunnel syndrome during and after pregnancy. *Muscle Nerve* 2002;25:914–17
11. Courts RB. Splinting for symptoms of carpal tunnel syndrome during pregnancy. *J Hand Ther* 1995;8:31–4
12. Wood C. Paresthesia of the hand in pregnancy. *Br Med J* 1961;2:680–2
13. al Quattan MM, Manktelow RT, Bowen CVA. Pregnancy-induced carpal tunnel syndrome requiring surgical release longer than 2 years after delivery. *Obstet Gynecol* 1994;84:249–51
14. Donaldson JO. Pregnancy. In Evans RW, Basking DS, Yatsu PM, eds. *Prognosis of Neurological Disorders*. New York: Oxford University Press, 1992:673–9
15. Massey EW. Mononeuropathies in pregnancy. *Semin Neurol* 1988;8: 193–6
16. Racz GB, Hagstrom D. Iliohypogastric and ilioinguinal nerve entrapment: diagnosis and treatment. *Pain Digest* 1992;2:43–8
17. Carter BL, Racz GB. Iliohypogastric nerve entrapment in pregnancy: diagnosis and treatment. *Anesth Analg* 1994;79:1193–4
18. Bell C. Appendix. In Taylor J, ed. *The Nervous System of the Human Body*. London: Longman Rees Orme Brown, Gree, 1930:IV–V
19. Hilsinger RL, Adour KK, Doty HE. Idiopathic facial paralysis, pregnancy, and the menstrual cycle. *Ann Otol Rhinol Laryngol* 1975;84:433–42
20. Robinson JR, Pou JW. Bell's palsy. A predisposition of pregnant women. *Arch Otolaryngol* 1972;95:125–9
21. Cohen Y, Lavie O, Granovsky-Grisaru S, *et al.* Bell's palsy in pregnancy. *Obstet Gynecol Surv* 2000;55:184–8

22. Adour KK, Bell DN, Hilsinger RL. Herpes simplex virus in idiopathic facial paralysis (Bell's palsy). *J Am Med Assoc* 1975;233:527–30
23. Falco NA, Eriksson E. Idiopathic facial palsy in pregnancy and puerperium. *Surg Gynecol Obstet* 1989;169:337–40
24. Shmorgun D, Chan WS, Ray JG. Association between Bell's palsy in pregnancy and preeclampsia. *Q J Med* 2002;95:359–62
25. Walling AD. Bell's palsy in pregnancy and puerperium. *J Fam Pract* 1993; 36:559–63
26. McGregor JA, Guberman A, Amer J, Goodlin R. Idiopathic facial nerve paralysis (Bell's palsy) in late pregnancy and the early puerperium. *Obstet Gynecol* 1987;69:435–8
27. Gillman GS, Schaitkin BM, May M, *et al.* Bell's palsy in pregnancy: a study of recovery outcomes. *Otolaryngol Head Neck Surg* 2002;126:26–30
28. Wolf SM, Wagner JH, Davison S, Forsyth A. Treatment of Bell's palsy with prednisone: a prospective, randomized study. *Neurology* 1978;28: 158–61
29. Klein CJ, Dyck PJ, Friedenberg SM, *et al.* Inflammation and neuropathic attacks in hereditary brachial plexus neuropathy. *J Neurol Neurosurg Psychiatry* 2002;73:45–50
30. Simonetti S. Lesion of the anterior branch of the axillary nerve in a patient with hereditary neuropathy due to pressure palsies. *Eur J Neurol* 2000;7:577–9
31. Rihane B, LeBorghe JM, *et al.* Idiopathic brachial neuralgia after Caesarian section. *Ann Françaises Anesth Réanim* 2002;21:734–6
32. Hughes RA, Winer JB. Guillain–Barré syndrome. In Mathews WB, Glasser GH, eds. *Recent Advances in Clinical Neurology*. London: Churchill Livingstone, 1984:4
33. Ropper AH. The Guillain–Barré syndrome. *N Engl J Med* 1992;326: 1130–5
34. Clifton ER. Guillain–Barré syndrome, pregnancy, and plasmapheresis. *J Am Osteopath Assoc* 1992;92:1279–82
35. May SE, Causle MR, Kleinman GE. Landry–Guillain–Barré–Strohl syndrome in pregnancy: a report of two cases. *J Reprod Med* 1989;34:550–2
36. Hurley TU, Brunson AD, Archer RL, *et al.* Landry–Guillain–Barré–Strohl syndrome in pregnancy: report of three cases treated with plasmapheresis. *Obstet Gynecol* 1992;78:482–5
37. Bravo RH, Katz M, Inturrisi M, *et al.* Obstetric management of Landry–Guillain–Barré syndrome: a case report. *Am J Obstet Gynecol* 1982;142:714–15
38. Kuller JA, Katz VL, McCoy MC, *et al.* Pregnancy complicated by Guillain–Barré syndrome. *South Med J* 1995;88:987–9
39. Nesbitt I. Pregnancy, anesthesia and Guillain–Barré syndrome. *Anaesthesia* 2000;55:1227–8
40. Mendizabal JE, Bassam AB. Guillain–Barré syndrome and cytomegalovirus infection during pregnancy. *South Med J* 1997;90:63–4
41. Rockel A, Vissel J, Rolfs A. Guillain–Barré syndrome in pregnancy – an indication for Caesarian section? *J Perinat Med* 1994;22:393–8

42. Bolik A, Wissel J, Rolfs A. Guillain–Barré syndrome in pregnancy – two case reports and a discussion on management. *Arch Gynecol Obstet* 1995; 256:199–203
43. Graves G, Oates M. Therapeutic plasma exchange for Guillain–Barré syndrome during pregnancy. *ANNA J* 1994;21:277–8
44. Van der Meche FGA, Schmit PIM, for the Dutch Guillain–Barré Study Group. A randomized trial comparing intravenous immunoglobulin and plasma exchange in Guillain–Barré syndrome. *N Engl J Med* 1992;326: 1123–9
45. Branch D, Ware MD, Porter T, *et al*. Obstetric uses of intravenous immunoglobulin: success, failures, promises. *J Allergy Clin Immunol* 2001; 108(Suppl):S133–8
46. Dyck PJ, Lais AC, Ohta M, *et al*. Chronic inflammatory polyradiculoneuropathy. *Mayo Clin Proc* 1975;50:621–36
47. Dyck PJ, Prineas J, Pollard J. Chronic inflammatory demyelinating polyradiculoneuropathy. In Dyck PJ, Thomas PK, Griffin JW, *et al*., eds. *Peripheral Neuropathy*, 3rd edn. Philadelphia: WB Saunders, 1993: 1498–517
48. McCombe PA, McManis PG, Frith JA, *et al*. Chronic inflammatory demyelinating polyneuropathy associated with pregnancy. *Ann Neurol* 1981;21:102–4
49. Small GA, Lovelace RE. Chronic inflammatory demyelinating polyneuropathy. *Semin Neurol* 1993;13:305–12
50. American Academy of Pediatrics Committee on Drugs. Transfer of drugs and other chemicals into human milk. *Pediatrics* 1989;84:924–36
51. Schabel JE. Subarachnoid block for a patient with progressive chronic inflammatory demyelinating polyneuropathy. *Anesth Analg* 2001;93: 1304–6
52. Chaudhry V, Escolar DM, Cornblath DR. Worsening of multifocal motor neuropathy during pregnancy. *Neurology* 2002;59:139–41
53. Vital A, Larrivietre M, Lagueny AME, *et al*. Severe axonal polyneuropathy with onset in the postpartum period. *Acta Neurol Scand* 1994;89: 303–6
54. Watson WJ, Beebe J. Postpartum foot drop. *J Reprod Med* 1988;33:973–4
55. Reif ME. Bilateral common peroneal nerve palsy secondary to prolonged squatting in natural childbirth. *Birth* 1988;15:100–2
56. Colachis SC, Pease WS, Johnson EW. A preventable cause of foot drop during childbirth. *Am J Obstet Gynecol* 1994;171:270–2
57. Vargo MM, Robinson LR, Nicolas JJ, *et al*. Postpartum femoral neuropathy: a relic of an earlier era? *Arch Phys Med Rehab* 1990;71:591
58. Dar AQ, Robinson A, Lyons G. Postpartum femoral neuropathy: more common than you think. *Anaesthesia* 1999;54:512
59. Al Hakim M, Katirji MB. Femoral mononeuropathy induced by the lithotomy position: a report of 5 cases with review of literature. *Muscle Nerve* 1993;16:891–5
60. Kofler M, Kronenberg MF. Bilateral femoral neuropathy during pregnancy. *Muscle Nerve* 1988;21:1106
61. Wirz D, Mashman J. Bilateral postpartum femoral neuropathy. *Conn Med* 1985;49:496–8

62. Montag TW, Mead PB. Postpartum femoral neuropathy. *J Reprod Med* 1981;26:563–6
63. Kuntzer T, Melle GV, Regli F. Clinical and prognostic features in unilateral femoral neuropathies. *Muscle Nerve* 1997;20:205–11
64. Lindner A, Shulte-Mattler W, Zierz S. Post partal obturator neuropathy: case report and review of nerve compression syndromes during pregnancy and delivery. *Zentralbl Gynakol* 1997;119:93–9
65. Fitzpatrick M, O'Herlihy C. The effects of labor and delivery on the pelvic floor. *Best Pract Res Clin Obstet Gynaecol* 2001;15:63–79
66. Sultan AH, Kamm MA, Hudson CN. Pudendal nerve damage during labor: prospective study before and after childbirth. *Br J Obstet Gynaecol* 1994;101:22–8
67. Lee SJ, Park JW. Follow-up evaluation of the effect of vaginal delivery on the pelvic floor. *Dis Colon Rectum* 2000;43:1550–5
68. Blyaert A, Soetens M, Vaes L, *et al*. Bupivacaine, 0.125 per cent, in obstetric epidural analgesia: experience in three thousand cases. *Anesthesiology* 1979;52:435–8
69. Scott DB, Hibbard BM. Serious non-fatal complications associated with extradural block in obstetric practice. *Br J Anaesth* 1990;64:537–41
70. Kane RE. Neurological deficits following epidural or spinal anesthesia. *Anesth Analg* 1981;60:150–61
71. Moore DC, Bridenbaugh LD, Thomson GE, *et al*. Bupivacaine: a review of 11 080 cases. *Anesth Analg* 1978;57:42–53
72. Reynolds F. Damage to the conus medullaris following spinal anaesthesia. *Anesthesia* 2001;56:238–47
73. Biousse V, Guevara G, Newman N. Transient Horner's syndrome after lumbar epidural anesthesia. *Neurology* 1998;51:1473–5
74. Yuen E, Layzer R, Weitz S, *et al*. Neurologic complications of lumbar epidural anesthesia and analgesia. *Neurology* 1995;45:1795–8
75. Tsen L, Cherayil G. Sickle cell-induced peripheral neuropathy following spinal anesthesia for Cesarean delivery. *Anesthesiology* 2001;95:1298–9

7

Myasthenia gravis and pregnancy

E. Ciafaloni and J. M. Massey

INTRODUCTION

Myasthenia gravis

Myasthenia gravis (MG) is an acquired autoimmune disease in which pathogenic autoantibodies against the acetylcholine receptors (AChRs) at the neuromuscular junction induce failure of neuromuscular transmission, resulting in muscle fatigue and weakness.

The association of specific human leukocyte antigen (HLA) haplotypes in MG patients suggests a genetic susceptibility to develop the disease, but familial autoimmune MG is very rare. Onset of disease can occur at any age, but female incidence peaks in the third decade while male incidence is greatest in the sixth and seventh decades of life. Females are more common among the children and young adults affected by MG. The mean age at onset is 28 years in females and 42 years in males. The ratio of female/male patients is 6 : 4.

Patients present with fluctuating muscle weakness that increases with repeated or sustained exertion and during the course of the day, and improves with rest. The onset of symptoms can be acute or subacute, and relapses and remissions can occur. Onset and exacerbations can be precipitated by surgery, general anesthesia, infections, pregnancy and postpartum. The external ocular muscles are affected in the majority of patients, and ptosis and diplopia are common presenting symptoms. In about 20% of patients the symptoms remain limited to the ocular musculature (ocular MG). Limb, bulbar and respiratory muscles are affected in variable degrees and combinations, causing mild to severe limb weakness, dysarthria, dysphagia and shortness of breath. Fluctuation in the severity of symptoms and objective fatigability of muscle weakness are characteristic of MG, and aid in establishing the diagnosis. Fixed muscle weakness, particularly of ocular muscles, is present in longstanding or poorly controlled cases of the disease. Weakness is worsened by

Table 1 Drugs that may cause myasthenia gravis exacerbation

Aminoglycoside antibiotics
Other antibiotics: erythromycin, ciprofloxacin, azithromycin
Beta-blocking agents
Botulinum toxin
Interferon-α
Calcium channel blockers
Magnesium, magnesium salts contained in some laxatives and antacids
Quinine, quinidine, procainamide
Neuromuscular blocking agents such as succinylcholine, vecuronium, curare-like agents
Iodinated contrast agents
Penicillamine
Eye drops used in management of glaucoma: timolol, betaxolol hydrochloride, echothiophate

elevation of body temperature, infections, emotional upsets, menses, surgery and several drugs (Table 1). Exacerbations can be unpredictable. Myasthenic crises are life-threatening exacerbations characterized by acute respiratory or bulbar paralysis, frequently requiring mechanical ventilation. Cholinergic crises caused by overuse of anticholinesterase medications are characterized by worsening weakness accompanied by hypersalivation, miosis, sweating, vomiting, diarrhea and lacrimation, and need to be distinguished from myasthenic crises.

Myasthenia gravis is associated with other autoimmune diseases, including rheumatoid arthritis, systemic lupus erythematosus, pernicious anemia, polymyositis and vitiligo. Thyroid disease is associated with MG in 13% of patients and can worsen the disease if untreated.

The clinical diagnosis is confirmed by demonstrating the presence of serum AChR antibodies. Elevated titers are present in about 80% of patients with generalized MG and in about 50% of purely ocular cases, and therefore a negative test does not rule out the diagnosis. Antibody titers do not correlate well with disease severity. Antistriated muscle antibodies are frequently present in the serum of MG patients, and tend to be associated with thymoma and late-onset disease. It has recently been shown that about 70% of AChR antibody-negative MG patients have serum antibodies against the muscle-specific receptor tyrosine kinase (MuSK)[1]. The MuSK antibodies are not present in AChR antibody-seropositive MG patients or those with purely ocular muscle weakness, and seem to define an immunologically distinct subgroup of patients.

A decremental response of the compound action muscle potential on 3-Hz repetitive nerve stimulation test (>10%) or abnormal neuromuscular jitter with or without blocking on single-fiber electromyogram (SFEMG) help to confirm the diagnosis, and are especially important in seronegative cases. These electrodiagnostic tests should be performed in clinically weak muscles to increase their sensitivity.

Edrophonium (Tensilon®), a short-acting acetylcholine esterase inhibitor, is given intravenously to demonstrate improvement of muscle weakness and to support the diagnosis (Tensilon test). Unfortunately, false-negative and false-positive results are not unusual. When performing a Tensilon test, there is a small risk of inducing bradycardia and cardiac collapse, and, therefore, atropine should be available.

Thymus hyperplasia is present in 60–80% of all MG patients, and suggests a pathogenic role of the thymus in the breakdown of self-tolerance leading to MG. Most child-bearing women with MG have an enlarged thymus and detectable circulating AChR antibodies.

Thymus imaging by computerized tomography (CT) or magnetic resonance imaging (MRI) should be performed to exclude the presence of a thymoma. Thymomas are present in about 10% of MG patients, are more frequent over the age of 30 and are very rare in juvenile MG. In patients with thymoma, AChR antibodies are present, often with antistriated muscle antibodies. Patients with a thymic tumor develop MG in 30–60% of cases.

Thymectomy is mandatory in patients with thymoma, and recommended in patients below age 50 with generalized MG. Thymectomy is usually not beneficial in late-onset MG, and it is very rarely done in purely ocular cases. Remission is possible in about 40–50% of cases.

Oral anticholinesterase agents such as pyridostigmine (Mestinon®) are used as symptomatic treatment while immunosuppressants such as corticosteroids, azathioprine, mycophenolate mofetil and cyclosporin are used for long-term treatment. Methotrexate and cyclophosphamide are used in more refractory cases. Plasmapheresis and intravenous immunoglobulin (IVIG) are used for acute treatment of MG exacerbations and myasthenic crises, to optimize perioperative management prior to thymectomy or other major surgeries and in severe cases refractory to all immunosuppressants.

Issues in the care of women with myasthenia gravis

As with a number of autoimmune diseases, MG occurs commonly in young women in their child-bearing years. The occurrence of MG in women poses several unique issues related to treatment. Severe generalized weakness and, in particular, respiratory insufficiency may endanger both mother and fetus. Medications used to control the MG symptoms must be thoughtfully chosen with consideration of their possible effect on the fetus, the pregnancy and the mother. Successful management of MG during pregnancy and in the postpartum period requires collaboration between the obstetrician and the neurologist. Women with MG should discuss their plan for pregnancy with their neurologist early on. The neurologist and obstetrician should be able to discuss treatment options and pregnancy risks based on the best current knowledge, so that women will be able to make an informed decision and successfully complete pregnancy.

MATERNAL MYASTHENIA AND THE RISKS TO NEWBORNS

Transient neonatal myasthenia gravis

Transient neonatal MG (NMG) occurs in about 10–20% of newborns of myasthenic mothers, and is caused by transplacental passive transfer of circulating AChR antibodies from the myasthenic mother to the fetus[2–6]. It is not possible to predict correctly the occurrence and severity of NMG. The clinical severity of MG symptoms in the mother does not correlate with severity in the newborn, and NMG has been reported in infants of myasthenic mothers who were in clinical remission. In general, a correlation between the occurrence and severity of NMG and overall high AChR antibody titers in the mothers as well as in the newborns has been observed; however, exceptions are not infrequent, and antibody titer cannot be considered an absolute marker for NMG as other factors in the fetal environment may play an important role in the clinical manifestation of NMG. Even some myasthenic women without elevated AChR antibodies have had babies with NMG[7,8]. A close correlation has been found between the occurrence of NMG and a high ratio of antifetal AChR to antiadult muscle AChR antibodies[9,10].

Symptoms develop in the first few hours after birth (12–48 h), and include difficulty feeding, respiratory distress, feeble cry, ptosis, facial paresis and generalized weakness and hypotonia. The severity of symptoms varies from child to child, with some showing only mild hypotonia and others having respiratory distress severe enough to require assisted ventilation. The delayed onset of NMG is attributed to the possible transfer of water-soluble anticholinesterase medications from the mother, and to the inhibitory effect of α-fetoprotein (AFP) on the anti-AChR antibodies. AFP has a powerful inhibitory effect on AChR antibody binding capacity, and high AFP levels may therefore protect the majority of newborns from developing clinical NMG[11,12]. The symptoms respond to anticholinesterase medications, and progressively improve as the antibody titer gradually falls. The syndrome usually resolves within a few weeks (18–21 days), but can occasionally persist for as long as 4 months. Every newborn of myasthenic mothers should be closely monitored during the first few days postpartum for signs of muscular weakness, especially affecting swallowing and respiratory muscles. Anticholinesterase drugs and ventilatory support should be used until the weakness resolves. Plasmapheresis in very severe cases may be considered.

Arthrogryposis

Arthrogryposis multiplex congenita (AMC) consists of non-progressive multiple congenital joint contractures developing *in utero* from lack of fetal movement preventing normal joint formation. AMC can lead to intrauterine or neonatal death due to pulmonary hypoplasia and polyhydramnios. Some cases are genetically determined, and others derive from primary muscle problems or lack of anterior horn cells. Maternal MG is a rare cause of AMC, and placental transfer of antibodies against the fetal AChR has been implicated as a possible cause[13–15]. Recurrent cases in sibships have been reported, even in initially asymptomatic mothers[16]. Some infants born with AMC from myasthenic mothers have survived, while others have died during the neonatal period or early infancy. A more complex phenotype including dysmorphic facies, abnormal genitalia, central nervous system atrophy and lung hypoplasia has also been reported in offspring born with AMC from MG mothers. Ultrasound evaluations should be used to monitor fetal movements and to detect the development of joint contractures *in utero*.

When counseling MG mothers, AMC and its high risk of recurrence need to be discussed among the possible complications. It should also be emphasized that the absence of MG symptoms in the mother does not guarantee the birth of a normal newborn. The potential role of plasmapheresis and immunosuppression during early pregnancy in preventing the occurrence of AMC and improving the outcome of newborns is not known[17].

Obstetric complications and management of labor and delivery

An increase in pregnancy wastage and premature labor has been described in MG[5]. In his large 1991 literature review of 322 pregnancies in 225 myasthenic mothers, Plauche reported a perinatal mortality of approximately 68/1000 births, five times that of uncomplicated pregnancy. In this review series there were 276 live births (85.6%) and 14 spontaneous and 24 induced abortions for a total abortion rate of 11.8%. An increased prevalence of premature delivery in myasthenic pregnancy defined as less than 36 completed weeks or 2500 g has been reported to be as high as 36.5%[5]. In the more recent series of Batocchi and colleagues, 64 pregnancies in 47 myasthenic women were reported. There were ten abortions, three spontaneous (4.6%), four premature births (7.4%), one perinatal death and one fetal anomaly[18]. Preterm delivery owing to premature rupture of the membranes has been reported in myasthenic mothers taking corticosteroids.

While spontaneous abortions have been reported to produce clinical improvement of myasthenic exacerbation, there is no evidence that therapeutic pregnancy termination has a beneficial role in improving myasthenic symptoms occurring in the first trimester, and in fact exacerbations can be triggered by the anesthesia and surgical procedure[19–21].

The course of labor in myasthenic patients does not change, although shortened labors have been reported owing to generalized relaxation. MG does not have a deleterious effect on the uterine smooth muscle, and therefore the first stage of labor is not compromised. Striated muscles involved in the second stage of labor are at risk for easy fatigue because of the abnormal neuromuscular transmission, and therefore the physician should be prepared to assist the tired patient with outlet forceps or vacuum extraction if needed. Cholinesterase inhibitor medications should be administered parenterally during labor owing to unpredictable gastric absorption. It is better to use neostigmine, as pyridostigmine can cause sterile abscess. Neostigmine 1.5 mg for intramuscular or 0.5 mg for intravenous dosing each is equivalent to oral pyridostigmine 60 mg.

Myasthenic patients are very sensitive to many anesthetic agents, and epidural anesthesia is preferred in both vaginal and operative delivery. Pre-anesthetic evaluation including pulmonary function evaluation should be emphasized. Non-depolarizing muscle relaxants may induce an exaggerated or prolonged response, and should be avoided if possible. Careful post-anesthetic monitoring in an intensive-care unit setting is recommended. Physicians managing myasthenic women also should be aware of the risk posed by magnesium sulfate used for management of eclampsia, because of its interference with neuromuscular transmission.

Cesarean section can induce exacerbation, and should be performed exclusively based on obstetric indications.

Maternal myasthenia gravis therapy and its effects on the newborn and lactation

Patients with MG planning to become pregnant should seek counseling early, to maximize their clinical improvement prior to pregnancy and reach an informed decision regarding management of their disease during pregnancy. The risks and benefits of continuing versus discontinuing or decreasing immunosuppressant medications should be discussed, and recommendation should be based on the severity of MG and the presence of bulbar and respiratory weakness. In general, immunosuppressant medications should be discontinued or decreased to a minimum when disease severity allows, to avoid potential adverse effects on the fetus. However, the risk posed to both fetus and mother by uncontrolled MG and life-threatening exacerbation caused by immunosuppressant drug withdrawal needs to be carefully considered before any decision is made.

Pyridostigmine bromide (Mestinon), when used at the recommended dose of less than 600 mg/day, is considered safe during pregnancy. The frequency of malformations is not increased among the offspring of rats treated during pregnancy with various doses of pyridostigmine in a range similar to that used in humans[22]. An infant whose mother was taking 1500–3000 mg/day (4–8 times the recommended dose) of pyridostigmine bromide during pregnancy was born with severe NMG, growth restriction microcephaly, joint contractures and multiple dysmorphic features[23]. Intravenous cholinesterase inhibitors should be avoided, as premature labor may rarely occur.

The American Academy of Pediatrics classified pyridostigmine as compatible with breast-feeding. Large doses of anticholinesterase drugs may cause gastrointestinal upsets in the breast-fed newborn[24].

Plasmapheresis and IVIG can be effective and safe treatments for severe weakness or crises during pregnancy[25]. There is a theoretical risk that plasmapheresis may induce premature delivery because of the removal of circulating hormones[26]. Hypotension must be carefully monitored and corrected during the exchanges.

Hyperviscosity and volume overloading associated with IVIG may be of greater significance in pregnancy. Complications associated with IVIG use include stroke, renal failure, aseptic meningitis and hepatitis C[27].

There are few data available regarding the safety of immunosuppressant drugs in MG patients during pregnancy, and most information is derived from patients with other autoimmune diseases (inflammatory bowel disease, systemic lupus erythematosus, autoimmune hepatitis) and transplant recipients. In most available human studies it is frequently impossible to separate the effects of immunosuppressant drugs from the effects of other independent risk factors, such as the underlying maternal illness and concomitant use of other drugs.

Corticosteroid therapy presents little if any teratogenic risk to the fetus, and only a slight increase in the incidence of cleft palate has been reported[28]. Preterm delivery due to premature rupture of the membranes of an infant with respiratory distress and bacterial pneumonia, and one delivery of a boy with multiple congenital anomalies, have been reported[18,29,30]. Premature rupture of the membranes may be related to high-dose corticosteroid treatment. It is not clear whether either maternal or fetal risk of infection is increased with this therapy. Corticosteroids can be used safely during lactation[24].

Women with MG taking azathioprine have generally been advised against pregnancy, although there has never been definite demonstration of teratogenicity in humans at therapeutic doses, and many normal pregnancies have been reported while on the drug. Batocchi and colleagues reported in their series four MG patients who were taking azathioprine during pregnancy, and all of them gave birth to normal babies. In one patient the sudden withdrawal of azathioprine had no effect on the MG course, while it induced severe exacerbation of MG symptoms in another[18]. Azathioprine has been reported to be safe during pregnancy in inflammatory bowel disease[31]. During 40 years' experience with azathioprine as an immunosuppressant in organ transplant patients, the National Transplantation Pregnancy Registry has identified no predominant or specific fetal malformation pattern which is attributable to this drug, and the epidemiologic data available to date are favorable in the setting of a category D agent[32]. A retrospective review of pregnancy outcome revealed that infants exposed to azathioprine might develop reversible leukopenia, anemia, thrombocytopenia, reduced immunoglobulin levels, infection and thymic atrophy[33]. Babies born to mothers receiving azathioprine have an increased risk of myelosuppression and immunosuppression[34–36]. Breast-feeding is contraindicated in mothers receiving azathioprine[37].

Cyclosporin does not appear to be a major human teratogen, but seems to carry a higher risk of spontaneous abortions, prematurity and low birth weight.

The rate of low birth weight in cyclosporin-exposed pregnancies is increased over the rate in pregnancies in transplanted women who are not on cyclosporin (49% vs. 38%). Prematurity is not increased by cyclosporin exposure[32]. There was no evidence of nephrotoxicity in 26 children followed to an average age of 39 months after their birth to women who had been treated with cyclosporin during pregnancy[38]. Transient neonatal thrombocytopenia, neutropenia and lymphopenia have occasionally been reported in the infants of women treated with cyclosporin during pregnancy. Abnormalities of various lymphocyte subpopulations have been observed among such children up to 6 years after birth, although it is uncertain whether these alterations are of clinical importance. Cyclosporin is transferred to the breast milk. Some clinicians have recommended against breast-feeding while using this drug; however, others have reported successful breast-feeding while mothers were taking cyclosporin. Estimates of neonatal exposure to cyclosporin in breast milk indicate that it is likely to be far less than the levels to which the fetus had been exposed prenatally. In a group of seven infants breast-fed by mothers receiving cyclosporin A, it was estimated that the infants ingested less than 300 μg per day of cyclosporin A, and all infant blood levels were below 30 ng/ml, the detection limit of the drug assay[39]. There are no demonstrable nephrotoxic effects or other side-effects in infants exposed to cyclosporin in breast milk[39]. In a single case report, cyclosporin levels were undetectable in a neonate at various times during 10.5 months of exclusive breast-feeding from a woman on cyclosporin therapy[40].

Mycophenolate mofetil (MMF), in doses equivalent to those used clinically in transplant patients, caused fetal resorptions and malformations in pregnant rats and rabbits consisting predominantly of defects of the head and eyes. These malformations were found in the absence of maternal toxicity. Experience in transplant patients is still very limited, as MMF is a newer agent[41]. Only six reports of live births to female patients taking MMF have been reported to the National Transplantation Pregnancy Registry; none of these reports found major malformations in the offspring, but all were born prematurely. The only possible teratogenic effects detected were hypoplastic nails and short fifth fingers in one newborn of a mother who received a kidney transplant during the first trimester of pregnancy and took MMF, tacrolimus and prednisone for prevention of organ rejection. MMF should not be used in pregnancy until more information becomes available.

Methotrexate is a folic acid antagonist and should not be used to treat MG women of child-bearing age because of its association with congenital malformations, especially involving the central nervous system[42].

Methotrexate is excreted in breast milk in small quantities. Although the amount of methotrexate ingested daily through milk would be less than 0.5% of the pediatric therapeutic dose of this drug (0.12 mg/kg), the American Academy of Pediatrics listed methotrexate as being contraindicated during breast-feeding, and the World Health Organization Working Group on Drugs and Human Lactation did not recommend breast-feeding during the maternal use of this drug, unless no other alternative was available[37].

EFFECT OF PREGNANCY ON THE COURSE OF MYSASTHENIA GRAVIS

The course of MG may change during pregnancy, frequently in an unpredictable fashion. Approximately one-third of women worsen during this time. The worsening may occur at any time, but is more likely in the first trimester followed by improvement in the last two trimesters. Complete remission of MG symptoms may also occur during late pregnancy and may be followed by rapid postpartum exacerbation.

The first 3 weeks postpartum are particularly risky for sudden exacerbation, including respiratory insufficiency, and therefore careful monitoring and adequate therapy are necessary. Clinical state at the time of pregnancy does not predict the occurrence of exacerbation or remission. SFEMG has demonstrated changes that parallel the clinical fluctuations during pregnancy[43]. New onset of MG may occur in pregnancy or in the immediate postpartum. The mortality risk of myasthenic mothers seems to be inversely correlated with the duration of the disease, the highest risk being in the first year and minimal risk 7 years after onset of the disease[44].

Knowledge of the potential effect of pregnancy on the course of MG is limited, and based mostly on retrospective reports of single or low-number cases[5,18,45,46]. In 1955, Osserman reported 33 pregnancies in 22 myasthenic women: an exacerbation occurred in one-third while no change or remission occurred in the other two-thirds[45]. In Plauche's large literature review series of 322 pregnancies in 225 myasthenic mothers, exacerbations were reported in 41% during gestation and 29.8% in the puerperium. In 31.7% of pregnancies there were no changes in MG symptoms throughout gestation and the postpartum period. Maternal deaths were reported in nine cases, usually due to myasthenic crises. In one case the patient had received magnesium sulfate for pre-eclampsia[5]. Such reviews of the literature are obviously biased by the inclusion of case reports focusing on myasthenic pregnancies with complications or crises.

A more recent series from Italy reported 64 pregnancies in 47 myasthenic mothers from 1978 to 1997[18]. A clinical worsening occurred in 19%, improvement in 22% and no change in 59%. No correlation was found between MG severity before conception and exacerbation of symptoms during pregnancy. The clinical course of the disease during one pregnancy did not predict the course during a subsequent pregnancy, and the first trimester of pregnancy and the first month postpartum were the most critical periods for MG exacerbations[18].

Djelmis and colleagues described 69 pregnancies in 65 myasthenic women and showed that MG symptoms worsened in 15% during pregnancy and a further 16% in the puerperium[46]. All women with puerperal infections developed exacerbations. The duration of MG was statistically shorter in the women who developed exacerbation in the postpartum period. The mode of delivery seemed not to affect the incidence of an exacerbation during the puerperium[46].

CONCLUSIONS

The peak of onset of MG in women is during their child-bearing years. Women with MG and their physicians are faced with a number of difficult decisions regarding proceeding with pregnancy and treatment of MG during pregnancy and breast-feeding. Many unanswered questions remain regarding choice of therapy and its effect on the fetus, and even the effect on the pregnancy. Key features of optimal care for the MG mother include planning the pregnancy, rational choice of therapy aimed at protecting the mother, the fetus and the pregnancy, and close follow-up by a medical team.

References

1. Hoch W, McConville J, Melms A, *et al.* Autoantibodies to the receptor tyrosine kinase MuSK in patients with myasthenia gravis without acetylcholine receptor antibodies. *Nat Med* 2001;7:365–8
2. Donaldson JO, Penn AS, Lisak RP, *et al.* Antiacetylcholine receptor antibody in neonatal myasthenia gravis. *Am J Dis Child* 1981;135:222–5
3. Barlow CF. Neonatal myasthenia gravis. *Am J Dis Child* 1981;135:209
4. Plauche WC. Myasthenia gravis. *Clin Obstet Gynecol* 1983;26:592–604
5. Plauche WC. Myasthenia gravis in mothers and their newborns. *Clin Obstet Gynecol* 1991;34:82–99
6. Bartoccioni E, Evoli A, Casali C, *et al.* Neonatal myasthenia gravis: clinical and immunological study of seven mothers and their newborn infants. *J Neuroimmunol* 1986;12:155
7. Melber D. Maternal–fetal transmission of myasthenia gravis with negative acetylcholine receptor antibody. *N Eng J Med* 1988;318:996
8. Heckmatt JZ, Placzek M, Thompson AH, *et al.* An unusual case of neonatal myasthenia. *J Child Neurol* 1987;2:63
9. Gardnerova M, Eymard B, Morel E, *et al.* The fetal/adult acetylcholine receptor ratio in mothers with myasthenia gravis as a marker for transfer of the disease to the newborn. *Neurology* 1997;48:50–4
10. Vernet-der Garabedian B, Lacokova M, Eymard B, *et al.* Association of neonatal myasthenia gravis with antibodies against the fetal acetylcholine receptor. *J Clin Invest* 1994;94:555–9
11. Brenner T, Beyth Y, Abramsky O. Inhibitory effect of α-fetoprotein on the binding of myasthenia gravis antibody to acetylcholine receptor. *Proc Natl Acad Sci USA* 1980;77:3635–9
12. Hatada Y, Munemura M, Matsuo I, *et al.* Myasthenic crisis in the puerperium: the possible importance of α-fetoprotein: case report. *Br J Obstet Gynaecol* 1987;94:480
13. Vincent A, Newland C, Brueton L, *et al.* Arthrogryposis multiplex congenita with maternal antibodies specific for a fetal antigen. *Lancet* 1995;346:24–5
14. Riemersma S, Vincent A, Beeson D, *et al.* Association of arthrogryposis multiplex congenita with maternal antibodies inhibiting fetal acetylcholine receptor function. *J Clin Invest* 1996;98:2358–63
15. Polizzi A, Huson S, Vincent A. Teratogen update: maternal myasthenia gravis as a cause of congenital arthrogryposis. *Teratology* 2000;62:332–41

16. Barnes PRJ, Kanabar L, Brueton L, *et al.* Recurrent congenital arthrogryposis leading to a diagnosis of myasthenia gravis in an initially asymptomatic mother. *Neuromusc Dis* 1995;5:59–65
17. Carr SR, Gilchrist JM, Abuelo DN, *et al.* Treatment of antenatal myasthenia gravis. *Obstet Gynecol* 1991;78:485–9
18. Batocchi AP, Majolini L, Evoli A, *et al.* Course and treatment of myasthenia gravis during pregnancy. *Neurology* 1999;52:447–52
19. Hay DM. Myasthenia gravis in pregnancy. *Br J Obstet Gynaecol* 1969;76: 323
20. Kosovsky N, Spurt H, Osserman KE. Pregnancy in myasthenia gravis: discussion. *Am J Med* 1955;19:718
21. Viets HR, Schwab RS, Brazier JAB. The effects of pregnancy on the course of myasthenia gravis. *J Am Med Assoc* 1942;119:23–36
22. Levine BS, Parker RM. Reproductive and developmental toxicity studies of pyridostigmine bromide in rats. *Toxicology* 1991;69:291–300
23. Niesen C, Shah NS. Pyridostigmine-induced microcephaly. *Neurology* 2000;54:1873–4
24. Committee on Drugs, American Academy of Pediatrics. The transfer of drugs and other chemicals into human breast milk. *Pediatrics* 1994;93: 137–50
25. Watson WJ, Katz VL, Bowes WA. Plasmapheresis during pregnancy. *Obstet Gynecol* 1984;76:451–7
26. Samuels P, Pfeifer SM. Autoimmune diseases in pregnancy. The obstetrician's view. *Rheum Dis Clin North Am* 1989;15:307–22
27. Kaaja R, Julkunen H, Ammala P, *et al.* Intravenous immunoglobulin treatment of pregnant patients with recurrent pregnancy losses associated with antiphospholipid antibodies. *Acta Obtet Gynecol Scand* 1993;72: 63–6
28. Fraser FC, Sajoo A. Teratogenic potential of corticosteroids in humans. *Teratology* 1995;51:45–6
29. Gaudier FL, Santiago-Delin E, Rivera J, *et al.* Pregnancy after renal transplantation. *Surg Gynecol Obstet* 1988;167:533–43
30. Schmidt PL, Sims ME, Strassner HT, *et al.* Effect of antepartum glucocorticoid administration upon neonatal respiratory distress syndrome and perinatal infection. *Am J Obstet Gynecol* 1984;178:178–86
31. Alstead EM, Ritchie JK, Lennard-Jones JE, *et al.* Safety of azathioprine in pregnancy in inflammatory bowel disease. *Gastroenterology* 1990;99: 443–6
32. Armenti VT, Radomski JS, Moritz MJ, *et al.* Report from the National Transplantation Pregnancy Registry (NTPR): outcomes of pregnancy after transplantation. *Clin Transpl* 2001;97:105
33. Armenti VT, Moritz MJ, Davison JM. Drug safety issues in pregnancy following transplantation and immunosuppression: effects and outcomes. *Drug Safety* 1998;19:219–32
34. Davison JM, Dellagrammatikas H, Parkin JM, *et al.* Maternal azathioprine therapy and depressed hemopoiesis in the babies of renal allograft patients. *Br J Obstet Gynaecol* 1985;92:233–9

35. DeWitte DB, Buick MK, Cyran SE, *et al.* Neonatal pancytopenia and severe combined immunodeficiency associated with antenatal administration of azathioprine and prednisone. *J Pediatr* 1984;105:625–8
36. Heneghan MA, Norris SM, O'Grady JG, *et al.* Management and outcome of pregnancy in autoimmune hepatitis. *Gut* 2001;48:97–102
37. World Health Organization Working Group. In Bennet PN, ed. *Drugs and Human Lactation*. Amsterdam: Elsevier, 1988:369–70
38. Shaheen FAM, Al-Sulaiman MH, Al-Khadar AA. Long term nephrotoxicity after exposure to cyclosporine *in utero*. *Transplantation* 1993;56: 224–5
39. Nyberg G, Haljamae U, Frisenette-Fich C, *et al.* Successful beast-feeding during treatment with cyclosporine. *Transplantation* 1998;65:253–5
40. Munoz-Flores-Thiagarajan KD, Easterling T, Davis C, *et al.* Breast feeding by a cyclosporine-treated mother. *Obstet Gynecol* 2001;97:816–18
41. Pergola P, Kancharla A, Riley D. Kidney transplantation during the first trimester of pregnancy: immunosuppression with mycophenolate mofetil, tacrolimus, and prednisone. *Transplantation* 2001;71:994–7
42. Buckley LM, Bullaboy CA, Leichtman L, *et al.* Multiple congenital anomalies associated with weekly low-dose methotrexate treatment of the mother. *Arthritis Rheum* 1997;40:971–3
43. Massey JM, Sanders DB. Single fiber electromyography in myasthenia gravis during pregnancy. *Muscle Nerve* 1993;16:458–60
44. Scott JS. Immunologic diseases in pregnancy. *Prog Allergy* 1977;23:371–5
45. Osserman KE. Pregnancy in myasthenia gravis and neonatal myasthenia gravis. *Am J Med* 1955;19:718–21
46. Djelmis J, Sostarko M, Mayer D, *et al.* Myasthenia gravis in pregnancy: report on 69 cases. *Eur J Obstet Gynecol Reprod Biol* 2002;104:21–5

8

Central nervous system infections during pregnancy

C. B. Britton

INTRODUCTION

Central nervous system (CNS) infections rarely complicate pregnancy, but may be devastating for the mother and child when they occur. Prompt diagnosis and appropriate treatment are important for optimal maternal/fetal outcome. For transmissible infections, the health of the spouse or sexual partner as well as household and community contacts may also be at risk. Maternal treatment guidelines and maternal/fetal outcome data from population-based studies or large clinical trials are available for human immunodeficiency virus (HIV) infection, *Mycobacterium tuberculosis*, toxoplasmosis and Lyme disease. For most infections, the data on maternal/fetal outcomes and response to treatment are anecdotal, based on isolated case reports. Viral, bacterial, fungal and tuberculous infections are discussed.

GENERAL CONSIDERATIONS

The profound immunologic changes of pregnancy include the induction of T-cell tolerance to permit fetal development without rejection[1]. There is a theoretical risk that these changes could result in enhanced susceptibility to infection in pregnancy. In general, there is no evidence that the altered immune state of pregnancy changes susceptibility to infection, clinical symptomatology or treatment outcome. An exception is *Listeria* where pregnancy is considered a risk condition. Vaginal tract infectious colonization during pregnancy, e.g. with group B streptococcus, poses a risk to the fetus for intrapartum infection and a rare risk of maternal invasive disease and CNS involvement. Fungal infections acquired in the last trimester of pregnancy may more readily disseminate and involve the CNS.

Antimicrobial efficacy is largely unaltered by pregnancy, but treatment decisions are appropriately influenced by concern for fetal health. In some cases, maternal health cannot be restored without using drugs that may cause fetal harm. However, untreated infection risks both maternal and fetal well-being, so the best available treatment must be offered and the patient given information necessary for informed choice, including pregnancy termination, for early pregnancy where exposure to a potential teratogen is unavoidable, or where serious fetal abnormality is demonstrated due to infection or drug.

CNS infections may be discussed according to the clinical syndrome, e.g. meningitis, encephalitis, abscess or empyema, cord compression, myelitis, neuritis, or by the clinical course, e.g. acute, subacute, chronic, recurrent, or the pathogenic cause, e.g. virus, bacteria, fungus and protozoa. The clinical course is defined as follows: acute, symptoms less than 3 days; subacute, symptoms 3 days to 1 week; chronic, 1 week or more; recurrent, discrete events terminating spontaneously or after treatment.

Meningitis is a clinical syndrome of fever, headache, nuchal rigidity and variable impairment of consciousness, dependent on causative organism[2]. Photophobia, phonophobia, malaise, nausea and vomiting may also be present. Inflammatory cells and organisms are localized to the meninges without significant parenchymal involvement. Encephalitis is characterized by parenchymal involvement, indicated by focal signs, seizures and change in mental status. Meningoencephalitis combines clinical features of meningitis and encephalitis. Brain abscess or empyema is associated with severe headache, focal signs and sometimes seizures. Papilledema may be present.

Spinal cord empyema may cause cord compression and clinical signs of severe back pain, paraparesis or quadriparesis dependent on level, and bowel and bladder involvement. Myelitis is clinically similar to cord compression and may be incomplete or complete. Radiculitis refers to root pain, and if associated with spinal cord signs is termed myeloradiculitis, or, for peripheral nerve, radiculoneuritis. Neuritis may involve root, single or multiple nerves, and may be associated with spinal cord or root involvement.

MENINGITIS

Meningitis or meningoencephalitis is the most common clinical syndrome caused by infection of the nervous system. In adults, an aseptic or non-pyogenic etiology is more common than septic meningitis.

Aseptic or viral meningitis

Aseptic meningitis is typically of viral origin, but may be of non-infectious origin, e.g. tumor, inflammatory conditions (sarcoid, vasculitis, systemic lupus erythematosus), chemicals or medications. The term aseptic meningitis is also applied to a clinical and cerebrospinal fluid (CSF) profile that resembles that of viral origin but where a pathogen is later identified, e.g. *Mycoplasma*, bacteria such as *Nocardia* or *Listeria*, parasites and *Rickettsia*[2]. Parameningeal foci such as brain abscess or empyema and endocarditis are other potential causes of aseptic meningitis.

Clinically, this is a self-limited acute meningitis with mild to moderately severe symptoms of headache, fever and nuchal rigidity. Sensorium is clear or mildly altered. The CSF shows lymphocytic pleocytosis, normal glucose and normal or mildly elevated protein (protein maximum elevation <100 mg/dl). In exceptional cases, polymorphonuclear leukocytes are found in CSF examined early after symptom onset, and some viruses such as mumps may cause CSF glucose < 40 mg/dl (Table 1).

Enteroviruses cause more than half of the cases of viral or aseptic meningitis[6]. There are 64 serotypes that include the numbered enteroviruses, echoviruses, polio and Coxsackie viruses. Throat and rectal swab culture may suggest the diagnosis. The organism is infrequently cultured from CSF. Serologic confirmation of CSF infection is available at several state laboratories and the Centers for Disease Control and Prevention (CDC). Acute and 3–4-week interval convalescent serum should be assayed. Reverse-transcriptase polymerase chain reaction (RT-PCR) of CSF is both highly specific and sensitive for the diagnosis (Table 2)[8]. These viruses cross the placenta and adverse fetal outcomes are reported for Coxsackie virus[9].

Table 1 Cerebrospinal fluid (CSF) in meningitis[2–5]

	Acute		
CSF finding	*Bacterial*	*Viral*	*Chronic fungal/tuberculous*
Opening pressure	elevated	normal	elevated
White cell count	100–10 000	< 300	50–4000
Glucose	< 40 mg/dl	usually normal	< 40 mg/dl
Protein	100–500 mg/dl	usually normal	150 mg/dl to >1 g
Gram stain or smear	yes	no	India ink; acid-fast bacteria smear
Culture positive (%)	70–85	50	25–50/52–83

Table 2 Special studies in cerebrospinal fluid (CSF): antigen, endotoxin, antibody and polymerase chain reaction (PCR)[2–5,7]

Antigen and endotoxin tests
Steptococcus pneumoniae
*Neisseria meningitidis**
Group B streptococcus*
Haemophilus influenzae type H*
Cyptococcus neoformans
Gram-negative endotoxin

Antibody tests (serology)
Fungus
Coccidioides immitis
Histoplasma capsulatum
Candida albicans
Blastomyces dermatidis
Aspergillus
Sporothrix schenckii
Bacteria
VDRL; FTA-ABS
Brucella
Lyme ELISA and Western blot
Parasite
Taenia solium
Toxoplasma gondii

PCR assay
Herpes simplex type 1*
Cytomegalovirus
Varicella zoster virus*
Epstein–Barr virus*
Enterovirus*
Mycobacterium tuberculosis
Borrelia burgdorferi (Lyme)

*Indicates 100% specificity, sensitivity varies from 70% to near 100% for most organisms with highest sensitivity for *Cryptococcus* and Gram-negative endotoxin for antigen studies and herpes simplex virus, cytomegalovirus and enterovirus for PCR; VDRL, Venereal Disease Research Laboratory; FTA-ABS, fluorescent treponemal antibody absorption; ELISA, enzyme-linked immunosorbent assay

Viruses that typically cause encephalitis such as the herpes group viruses and arboviruses are infrequent causes of meningitis as well. A self-limited meningitis may be caused by genital herpes virus type 2. Other infrequent causes of meningitis include mumps and lymphocytic choriomeningitis.

Acute HIV infection may also cause aseptic meningitis at the time of initial exposure or seroconversion, and at any time during the course of infection. Initial serology may be negative, and should be repeated in 3 months in any case of aseptic meningitis. HIV serology should be routinely advised in pregnancy, and positive findings treated in accordance with accepted guidelines. It is well established that maternal treatment for HIV reduces the risk of fetal infection by 60% or more[10]. Treatment is usually begun after the first trimester of pregnancy. Fetal outcomes and early development appear to be normal after exposure to antiretroviral therapy, but long-term consequences of this drug exposure are not yet known.

The diagnosis of viral meningitis is one of exclusion, because the clinical and CSF profiles sometimes overlap those of bacterial infection. Empirical antibiotic and antiviral therapy for herpes simplex is usually indicated until cultures are reported as negative, but may be waived in very mild cases with normal CSF except for pleocytosis. Care is supportive and full recovery is expected.

Bacterial meningitis

Acute bacterial meningitis is a life-threatening medical emergency. Symptoms of fever, headache, confusion and nuchal rigidity evolve rapidly over hours in fulminant cases or over 2 or 3 days[11,12]. Clinical examination shows impaired mentation and stiff neck. Focal signs occurred in nearly 30% of patients in the Durand series and included seizures, cranial neuropathy or localized cerebral findings of aphasia or motor/sensory impairment[11]. Associated findings or conditions may include rash, sinusitis, mastoiditis, otitis media, endocarditis, pneumonia or liver disease. There is no evidence that pregnancy is a risk condition for bacterial meningitis since B-cell immunity is normal.

Lumbar puncture is diagnostic and should not be delayed[5]. Imaging studies are indicated before lumbar puncture when focal signs are present, but should not delay treatment. A magnetic resonance imaging (MRI) scan of the brain is preferred to computerized tomography (CT) in pregnancy to avoid fetal exposure to radiation, but may not always be feasible. Empirical treatment of meningitis without CSF examination risks inappropriate or delayed treatment for a non-bacterial pathogen. In the case that imaging is deemed necessary before lumbar puncture and will delay treatment, empirical therapy must be given. Gram stain and culture may become negative within hours of antibiotic therapy but other CSF abnormalities will persist for days or longer[8]. The CSF cell count may shift to a lymphocytic predominance on antibiotics.

CSF shows elevated opening pressure, moderate to marked pleocytosis, up to 20 000 white cells, predominantly polymorphonuclear

Table 3 Causes of bacterial meningitis, 1995, and treatment. Adapted from reference 13

Organism	*Incidence (cases/100 000)*	*Treatment*
Streptococcus pneumoniae	1.1	penicillin, cefotaxime or ceftriaxone
Neisseria meningitidis	0.6	penicillin, cefotaxime or ceftriaxone, rifampin
Group B streptococcus	0.3	penicillin or ampicillin
Listeria monocytogenes	0.2	ampicillin
Haemophilus influenzae	0.2	cefotaxime or ampicillin

cells, depressed glucose (< 40 mg/dl) and elevated protein, usual range 100–500 mg/dl (Table 1). CSF glucose should be compared with a simultaneous blood glucose; the normal ratio CSF/blood is 2 : 3. CSF Gram stain and culture are positive and diagnostic in more than 80% of cases. Blood cultures are usually positive as well. Polymerase chain reaction (PCR), bacterial antigen or endotoxin tests of CSF are helpful for partially treated meningitis (Table 2). For the pregnant patient, evaluation with blood cultures and lumbar puncture is appropriate, but radiographic studies should be avoided where possible, except for MRI, especially in the first trimester. A purified protein derivative (PPD) test with anergy panel and HIV serology are indicated in any patient with undiagnosed meningitis.

The development of a vaccine for *Haemophilus influenzae* resulted in the shift of bacterial meningitis from a disease of childhood to a disease of young adults with a median age of 25. A surveillance study of a defined geographic region of about 10 000 000 persons in the USA in 1995 yielded 248 cases of bacterial meningitis[13]. *Streptococcus pneumoniae* is the most common community-acquired pathogen, followed by *Neisseria meningitidis*, group B streptococcus, *Listeria* and *H. influenzae* (Table 3). There is epidemiologic evidence that African-Americans are at increased risk for septic meningitis. *Staphylococcus* and Gram-negative pathogens are common nosocomial pathogens, and occur in the setting of head trauma, neurosurgical procedures and immunosuppression. Group B streptococcus may cause bactiuria during pregnancy, and the more serious complication of amniotic infection with risk for maternal sepsis, rarely meningitis and intrauterine invasive fetal infection.

Empirical therapy of intravenous broad-spectrum antibiotics is based on epidemiologic considerations, Gram stain results if available and clinical findings[12,14–16]. The evaluation and treatment of the pregnant

Table 4 Food and Drug Administration (FDA) fetal risk categories* for antimicrobials commonly used in central nervous system infection[14,15]

Category B	*Category C*	*Category D*	*Category X*
Penicillins	carbapenems:	tetracycline	quinine
Cephalosporins	imipenem–cilastin	doxycylcine	
Meropenem	fluoroquinolones	streptomycin	
Clindamycin	trimethoprin–sulfamethoxazole		
Metronidazole	ganciclovir		
Gentamicin	foscarnet		
Vancomycin	mebendazole		
Aztreonam	mefloquine		
Erythromycin	chloroquine		
Azithromycin	primaquine		
Praziquantel	flucytosine		
Aciclovir	fluconazole		
Amphotericin B	itraconazole		
Ethambutol	rifampin		
	isoniazid		
	pyrazinamide		
	cycloserine		
	p-aminosalicylic acid		

*FDA category B, fetal risk not demonstrated in animal or human studies; category C, fetal risk unknown, no adequate human studies; category D, some evidence of fetal risk, may be necessary to use this drug; category X, proven fetal risk, contraindicated for use in pregnancy

patient does not differ from that of the non-pregnant patient except that, where possible, the Food and Drug Administration (FDA) fetal risk rating is considered (Table 4). A common initial therapy is penicillin or third-generation cephalosporin (cefotaxime or ceftriaxone) and ampicillin (Table 5). The cephalosporins are more often used if the organism is not known, pending culture. Vancomycin can be added to cover possible *Staphylococcus* infection or for penicillin-resistant *S. pneumoniae*, an increasing problem worldwide. Cefotaxime or ceftazidime should be combined with an aminoglycoside for suspected Gram-negative organisms. Oral rifampin is given for 2 days for *N. meningitidis*. Household and community contacts are similarly treated. Aciclovir is a reasonable addition to an empiric regimen when Gram stain is negative.

Severe cerebral edema and occasionally herniation may complicate bacterial meningitis. In this setting, lumbar puncture is relatively contraindicated, and measures to control cerebral edema are appropriate and include corticosteroids, intubation and hyperventilation. Other

Table 5 Antimicrobial dosage for central nervous system infection[3–5,14,15,17]

Antibacterials	
Ampicillin	2.0 g q4 h
Cefotaxime	2.0 g q6 h
Ceftriaxone	2.0 g q12 h
Ceftazidime	2.0 g q8 h
Gentamicin	2.0 mg/kg load, 1.7 mg/kg q8 h main (80 mg q8 h)
Meropenem	1.0 g q8h
Penicillin G	4.0 million units q4 h
Vancomycin	1.0 g q12 h
Antifungals	
Amphotericin B	0.3–0.7 mg/kg/day for 6 weeks to total dose of 1 to 2 g
Flucytosine	150 mg/kg/day in divided dose at 6-h intervals
Antivirals	
Aciclovir	10 mg/kg q8 h
Antituberculous drugs	
Isoniazid	300 mg/day po
Rifampin	600 mg/day po
Ethambutol	15–25 mg/kg/day po
Pyrazinamide	20–35 mg/kg/day po

q, every; po, by mouth

than for treatment of increased intracranial pressure, there is no evidence supporting routine use of corticosteroids in adult bacterial meningitis. Other potential complications are dementia, seizures, hydrocephalus, cerebral infarction, cerebral venous thrombosis, brain abscess or empyema.

For the young, outcome is related to the level of consciousness and presence of seizures at the time treatment is initiated. In the Durand analysis, there was 25% mortality for single-episode community-acquired meningitis and 35% mortality for single-episode nosocomial meningitis. There are no meaningful data on fetal outcome because of the rarity of bacterial meningitis in pregnancy, but normal outcomes are reported.

Listeria meningitis in pregnancy warrants special mention because pregnancy is considered a risk condition for listeriosis, especially in the third trimester[18]. Despite this, case reports of *Listeria* meningitis in pregnant women are rare. The organism is a food-borne pathogen acquired from coleslaw, contaminated pasteurized milk, Mexican-style soft cheese, ready-to-eat deli food, uncooked hot dogs, raw beef and poultry. Many cases, however, are sporadic without a recognized source.

The clinical presentation of *Listeria* meningitis is variable, and may be indolent with encephalopathy preceding meningeal signs by several days, resemble typical bacterial meningitis with fever, altered sensorium, seizures, meningeal and focal signs or resemble viral infection with malaise, gastrointestinal or flu-like symptoms and headache, sometimes with minimal meningeal signs on examination.

CSF findings may mimic those of viral meningitis with lymphocytic pleocytosis and normal glucose and protein. Early recognition and adequate treatment of the infection permit survival of the mother and child. When maternal listeriosis is unrecognized, severe fetal sequelae may ensue, including spontaneous abortion, prematurity, neonatal septic shock and death. Maternal death may also occur. Treatment is high-dose ampicillin and an aminoglycoside such as gentamicin for 3–4 weeks.

Lyme disease is a spirochetal infection caused by *Borrelia burgdorferi*, transmitted to humans by a deer tick, *Ixodes pacificus* in the western USA and *Ixodes scapularis* in the eastern USA[17]. More than 90% of cases are in ten states: Connecticut, Rhode Island, New Jersey, New York, Pennsylvania, Delaware, Massachusetts, Wisconsin, Minnesota and Maryland. The initial manifestation is a localized rash, erythema migrans. Hematogenous dissemination occurs early. Bell's palsy is an early neurologic symptom in Lyme disease, and may be bilateral. Neurologic complications of late Lyme include meningitis, myelitis and radiculoneuritis. Chronic encephalopathy with or without psychiatric features may occur. Leukoencephalitis similar to multiple sclerosis may also occur.

Transplacental transmission of *Borrelia* is established in humans and animals, and may result in disseminated infection in the fetus and fetal morbidity or death[19,20]. Although anecdotal case reports suggested that Lyme disease in pregnancy may be teratogenic, especially a cause of cardiac malformations, large prospective studies fail to show a teratogenic effect[21,22]. A prospective study of 2000 women showed no difference in fetal outcome for women exposed to Lyme just before or during pregnancy[23]. A fetal effect in women with remote exposure could not be excluded. A retrospective study of congenital heart disease found no association with maternal tick bite[24].

The CSF in Lyme meningitis resembles that of viral infection, predominantly lymphocytic pleocytosis, normal or moderately elevated protein and normal glucose. Serologic studies in blood and CSF establish a diagnosis of CNS Lyme, but false-negatives may occur. PCR of CSF is helpful when positive, but a negative result does not exclude the diagnosis (Table 2).

Peripheral manifestations of Lyme, Bell's palsy and peripheral neuropathy, may be treated with oral antibiotics. Doxycycline, the standard therapy, is contraindicated in pregnancy. Erythromycin or penicillin may be used for peripheral manifestations. Two to four weeks of intravenous ceftriaxone is standard treatment for acute Lyme meningitis. Longer treatment regimens are often given if the illness is of long duration or if the response to treatment is slow. There is no consensus on the use of prophylactic antibiotics for an asymptomatic pregnant woman with a history of tick bite of short duration, although most clinicians might find it prudent to treat.

Borrelia species also cause relapsing fever where neurologic syndromes overlap those of Lyme, i.e. facial palsy and meningitis. Antibiotic treatment is similar.

Neurosyphilis is caused by *Treponema pallidum*. The incidence of primary and secondary syphilis rose with the spread of the acquired immune deficiency syndrome (AIDS) epidemic from the 1980s to the mid-1990s, and now appears to be leveling off in some populations in the USA[25]. Syphilis is a risk factor for HIV transmission. HIV serology is indicated in all who test positive for syphilis. The neurologic syndromes of syphilis are asymptomatic CSF pleocytosis, acute meningitis with or without cranial neuropathy and tabes dorsalis and general paresis, a chronic frontotemporal encephalitis causing dementia and psychiatric disturbances. Placental transmission and congenital infection are well-documented.

The CSF shows predominantly lymphocytic pleocytosis, normal glucose, mildly elevated protein and a positive CSF Venereal Disease Research Laboratory (VDRL) test. Uncommonly, CSF VDRL is negative in cases of neurosyphilis. In this case, a non-reactive CSF fluorescent treponemal antibody absorption test excludes the diagnosis[17].

High-dose intravenous penicillin for 10–14 days is the accepted treatment and will usually result in cure. Those dually infected with HIV and syphilis are at risk for relapse with ocular and CNS persistence of infection. The standard therapy is not altered, but patients should be closely followed and retreated if titers do not decline by at least two dilutions in 3 months. Some advocate lumbar puncture and more aggressive treatment of all HIV infected persons with primary and secondary syphilis, but there is no consensus that this is necessary.

Chronic meningitis

Clinical signs evolve slowly over days to weeks. Headache, confusion, cranial neuropathy, seizures and focal signs may occur. Fever may not be prominent. Tuberculosis, cryptococcosis and toxoplasmosis are the most common infectious causes of chronic meningitis, and may also cause brain abscess[4,13,26–29]. Cranial neuropathy is related to the characteristic basilar meningitis of tuberculosis and fungal infection. Cranial arteritis may also occur. Despite the role of T-cell immunity in these infections, there is no evidence that pregnancy alters the clinical presentation, outcome or response to treatment for these infections. Tuberculin reactivity and serological responses are unaffected by pregnancy. The risk of extrapulmonary tuberculosis is not increased by pregnancy.

CSF shows lymphocytic pleocytosis, depressed glucose and elevated protein in both tuberculosis and fungal infection (Table 1). Markedly elevated protein in tuberculosis (>1 g/dl) may indicate spinal block. CSF culture and PCR studies are helpful in the diagnosis of tuberculosis. CSF adenosine deaminase levels are elevated in tuberculosis. Cryptococcal antigen in blood and CSF and fungal cultures are diagnostic in almost all cases. Large-volume CSF culture (20–30 ml) enhances the chance for positive tuberculosis or fungal culture. Repeated lumbar punctures may be necessary for diagnosis. Enzyme-linked immunosorbent assay (ELISA) serology in serum and CSF and PCR of CSF may be helpful for the diagnosis of toxoplasmosis. When the clinical presentation is abscess, brain biopsy may be necessary, if serology and PCR are not diagnostic. MRI of brain in fungal or tuberculous meningitis may show intense basilar enhancement, abscess formation or hydrocephalus.

Tuberculosis in pregnancy should be promptly treated[29]. Perinatal transmission of tuberculosis from a mother with tuberculous meningitis to a child is reported[30]. First-line drugs for tuberculous meningitis include isoniazid, streptomycin, ethambutol, pyrazinamide and rifampin. Streptomycin is contraindicated in pregnancy because of otoxicity. No teratogenic effect in humans of the other first-line drugs has been demonstrated. There is concern about isoniazid maternal hepatotoxicity in pregnancy, however. Breast-feeding is not prohibited during treatment, but it is recommended that medications follow the first breast-feed and that a bottle be substituted for the first feed after medication.

There are several treatment regimens that range from 6 to 18 months' duration. Therapy is usually initiated with three drugs (isoniazid, rifampin and pyrazinamide) for 2 or 3 months with two-drug maintenance (isoniazid and rifampin) for 4–9 months or longer. Pyridoxine is given to prevent peripheral neuropathy due to isoniazid. Compliance is critical to prevent drug resistance. Concomitant infection with HIV does not alter treatment recommendations. Resistant organisms and atypical mycobacterium have been observed since the AIDS epidemic. Multidrug, protracted treatment is necessary.

Extrapulmonary tuberculosis in pregnancy is too rare to establish outcome statistics. Treatment may be successful for mother and child, if the disease is promptly diagnosed and treated. Corticosteroids are used as adjunctive therapy for the mass effect of tuberculomas or clinical deterioration sometimes observed on initiation of antimicrobial therapy. Sequelae may include hydrocephalus, cognitive impairment, seizures and visual impairment.

Disseminated fungal infection with meningitis is reported in pregnancy. Cryptococcal meningitis is most common, but coccidioidomycosis and blastomycosis CNS infections are reported[26,28,31,32]. Successful treatment with amphotericin B with and without flucytosine is described with no adverse impact on the fetus, including a few cases of first-trimester treatment. Maternal toxicity includes renal insufficiency, hypokalemia and anemia, all usually reversible on cessation of treatment. Amphotericin B is teratogenic in animal studies, but is FDA category B in humans owing to a low observed rate of adverse fetal effects (Tables 4 and 5). Flucytosine is FDA category C.

Oral therapy with fluconazole or itraconazole may successfully treat mild cases of meningitis, but both are teratogenic in animals, FDA category C in humans. An infant with malformations was noted in the first report of a pregnant woman treated with fluconazole[33]. Others have been treated with this class of antifungal with no adverse fetal effect. However, in view of the potential risk, these drugs are not recommended in pregnancy except where amphotericin cannot be given. Increased intracranial pressure should be aggressively treated to reduce mortality and morbidity. Corticosteroids, shunting and serial lumbar puncture to reduce CSF pressure may be used.

HIV serology is indicated in all patients with cryptococcal or other fungal infection. For *Cryptococcus*, response to therapy is monitored by lumbar puncture at 2 weeks for fungal culture and antigen determination. Persistent positive cultures or high antigen levels are associated with a poor prognosis. Duration of treatment of *Cryptococcus* with amphotericin is 4–6 weeks. In the immunosuppressed patient, oral fluconazole is continued thereafter, indefinitely, if there is no recovery or improvement in immunosuppression. For pregnant patients, this drug should be given after delivery. Breast-feeding should be avoided because of uncertain neonatal effects.

Coccidioidal meningitis also requires protracted therapy, for at least a year, and in some cases both intravenous and intrathecal administration of amphotericin[3]. Relapse rates are high, but are substantially reduced by long-term fluconazole therapy (200–400 mg/day). Potential sequelae of fungal meningitis include hydrocephalus, abscess formation, cerebral infarction, seizures and dementia.

ENCEPHALITIS

Herpes simplex is the most common cause of sporadic viral encephalitis. Symptoms and signs include fever, headache, altered sensorium, focal signs of language dysfunction or hemiparesis and seizures. CSF shows pleocytosis with early polymorphonuclear cells and later lymphocytic predominance, red cells, normal or moderately depressed glucose and mild-to-moderate protein elevation, usually less than 100 mg/dl. An electroencephalogram (EEG) may show frontal or temporal slowing and epileptiform discharges. MRI of the brain shows T2 hyperintensity in frontal and temporal regions. CT of these areas shows low-density lesions, sometimes with mass effect. Brain biopsy is diagnostic but is unnecessary because of the high sensitivity (100%) and specificity (100%) of CSF PCR for specimens collected within the first 10 days. Successful treatment of a pregnant woman with aciclovir and a good fetal outcome are reported[34].

Arboviruses cause sporadic and epidemic encephalitis, and include La Crosse (California group), St Louis, Japanese B, Eastern equine, Western equine and Venezuelan equine. Diagnosis is by acute and convalescent serologic studies in serum and CSF. Treatment is supportive. Ribavirin has been tried in La Crosse encephalitis. Mortality is variable, and ranges from 1% for Venezuelan equine to 50–75% for Eastern equine. West Nile virus is the most recently described arbovirus[35]. Of 3389 cases reported in 2002, meningoencephalitis occurred in 2354 or 69%. Intrauterine infection was recently reported in a woman with aseptic meningitis. The child had chorioretinitis and severe cerebral abnormalities[36].

Cytomegalovirus encephalitis is a consequence of disseminated cytomegalovirus (CMV) infection[37]. Risk conditions for this infection are advanced HIV and immunosuppression due to steroids or other drugs. Clinically, there is chronic progressive encephalopathy with cognitive and memory impairment with or without headache. Chorioretinitis may be present. Other clinical syndromes observed with this virus are myelitis and polyradiculopathy[38]. A unique aspect of this infection is the potential CSF finding of polymorphonuclear leukocyte predominance, especially in those with progressive polyradiculopathy. Blood or CSF cultures may be positive. Blood and CSF PCR studies are helpful if positive, but do not exclude the diagnosis if negative. CMV congenital infection may cause severe neurologic and other sequelae, or death. Ganciclovir and foscarnet are antivirals active against CMV. They are FDA category C drugs, but their use is necessary since disseminated CMV is life-threatening to mother and child.

Varicella zoster may cause localized skin eruption, localized encephalitis, myelitis and stroke[37]. Aciclovir is the treatment of choice. The risk of Epstein–Barr seroconversion in pregnancy is low[8,39]. Acute neurologic syndromes in adults are rare.

Malaria is a reportable disease in the USA[40]. This is a febrile illness with headache and constitutional symptoms that may rapidly progress to coma and death, if unrecognized. Cases are reported in American citizens, and foreign-born and military personnel. Malaria in pregnant women and congenital malaria are reported. The CDC advises women to avoid travel to malarious areas, if possible. Treatment recommendations are posted on their web site.

BRAIN ABSCESS

Bacterial brain abscess is rare in the general population and extremely rare in pregnancy. Risks for brain abscess are: penetrating head wound; contiguous source such as dental caries, sinusitis, otitis, mastoiditis, meningitis or osteomyelitis; endocarditis; and pleuropulmonary source. Alcoholism and intravenous drug use are important associated risk behaviors. Clinical symptoms and signs may include fever, headache, confusion, focal signs and seizures. Mixed aerobic and anaerobic pathogens are found at diagnostic brain biopsy. Medical cure with antibiotics is possible, reserving surgical intervention for large masses. Third-generation cephalosporins and metronidazole are usually given. Nafcillin is added for *Staphylococcus*.

Toxoplasmosis is the most common cause of brain abscess in AIDS, causing single or multiple abscesses with a predilection for the basal ganglia[41]. Empirical treatment with pyrimethamine and sulfadiazine is given for positive toxoplamosis serology, but should not be used before 17 weeks' gestation. Brain biopsy is considered for lesions that do not respond, or for serology-negative solitary lesions. If a mass effect does not preclude lumbar puncture, CSF PCR may be helpful[42].

Women with HIV infection may reactivate latent toxoplasmosis and acquire new infection during pregnancy[43,44]. Congenital transmission of both infections may occur with significant fetal morbidity or mortality[45]. There is no consensus on treatment, but some advocate spiramycin, a drug widely used in Europe, which concentrates in the placenta, and which can be used in the first trimester[46]. Treatment is continued throughout pregnancy.

In France, aggressive screening and treatment of pregnant women for toxoplasmosis is mandated by law[46]. There is no consistently applied guideline for diagnosis and treatment of this preventable infection in the USA. Preventive recommendations include: avoid contact with cat feces; wash fruits and vegetables before consumption; wash hands, kitchen utensils and surfaces after contact with uncooked meat or raw fruits and vegetables; cook meat to 150 °C before consumption; and prevent contamination of food by flies and cockroaches.

Cerebral cysticercosis is caused by eating uncooked or poorly cooked meat containing the cysts of *Taenia solium*[47]. Cysticercosis is a common cause of seizures in pregnancy in areas of central and Latin America. Encephalitis may also occur. Serologic studies of CSF and serum are helpful in diagnosis. MRI may show non-enhancing or enhancing cysts. Albendazole, the usual treatment for neurocysticercosis, is a category C drug in pregnancy, potentially teratogenic. If a patient is clinically stable with isolated seizures, anticonvulsants should be given and treatment deferred until delivery.

Subdural empyema and epidural abscess are both rare events. The clinical findings and associated risk conditions are similar to those of brain abscess. There are no specific data relating to pregnancy. These are life-threatening infections and should be managed similarly to those in the non-pregnant patient with surgical drainage and antibiotics.

SPINE AND SPINAL CORD INFECTIONS

Vertebral osteomyelitis and spinal epidural abscess are serious infections that are potential causes of irreversible spinal cord damage with paraplegia, and bowel and bladder involvement. Treatment is similar to that in the non-pregnant patient and may include surgical decompression and antibiotics. In some cases, immobilization with antibiotics is sufficient without the need for surgery[48]. Outcome depends on timely diagnosis and treatment. Organisms are usually cultured from blood.

Spinal cord intramedullary infection or myelitis is clinically similar, and may be due to virus (HIV, human T-cell leukemia virus-1 (HTLV-1), CMV, herpes simplex virus-2), toxoplasmosis or tuberculosis. Evaluation includes blood and CSF cultures for bacteria, fungus and viruses, PPD, HIV and HTLV-1 serology and MRI of the spine. Empirical antibiotic therapy should include coverage for Gram-negative organisms and *Staphylococcus* species, since trauma and drug use are often predisposing factors.

GUILLAIN–BARRÉ SYNDROME

Guillain–Barré syndrome (GBS) is an acute, monophasic inflammatory demyelinating polyneuropathy characterized by ascending paralysis, areflexia and albuminocytologic dissociation in the CSF. A similar syndrome with inflammatory cells in the CSF is termed acute inflammatory demyelinating polyneuropathy (AIDP). GBS and AIDP are associated with a number of infections that include *Campylobacter jejuni*, CMV, *Mycoplasma pneumoniae*, Epstein–Barr virus and HIV, among others.

Epidemiologic studies show that the risk of GBS is not altered by pregnancy but appears to be increased in the first 2 weeks postpartum[38,49–52]. Although maternal antibodies to peripheral nerve antigens were reported in one infant, there was no clinical impairment. Maternal treatment with intravenous immunoglobulin has been given successfully without adverse fetal consequence[7].

SUMMARY

Infections of the central nervous system are rare in pregnancy, and in general are evaluated and treated similarly to those in the non-pregnant patient, except that some medications and radiographic procedures are relatively contraindicated. Successful maternal/fetal outcome is dependent on timely diagnosis and treatment.

References

1. Mellor AL, Munn DH. Immunology at the maternal–fetal interface: lessons for T cell tolerance and suppression. *Annu Rev Immunol* 2000;18: 367–91
2. Coyle PK. Overview of acute and chronic meningitis. *Neurol Clin* 1999; 17:691–710
3. Davis LE. Fungal infections of the central nervous system. *Neurol Clin* 1999;17:761–81
4. Garcia-Monco JC. Central nervous system tuberculosis. *Neurol Clin* 1999; 17:737–60
5. Spach DH, Jackson LA. Bacterial meningitis. *Neurol Clin* 1999;17:711–35
6. Centers for Disease Control. Enterovirus surveillance – United States, 2000–2001. *Morbid Mortal Weekly Rep* 2002;51:1047–9
7. Yaneck H, Noro N, Kato EH, *et al*. Massive intravenous immunoglobulin treatment in pregnancy complicated by Guillain–Barré syndrome. *Eur J Obstet Gynecol Reprod Biol* 2001;97:101–4
8. Zunt JR, Marra CM. Cerebrospinal fluid testing for the diagnosis of central nervous system infection. *Neurol Clin* 1999;17:675–89
9. Euscher E, Davis J, Holzman I, Nuovo GJ. Coxsackie virus infection of the placenta associated with neurodevelopmental delays in the newborn. *Obstet Gynecol* 2001;98:1019–26
10. Mofenson LM. US Public Health Service task force recommendations for use of antiretroviral drugs in pregnant HIV-1 infected women for maternal health and interventions to reduce perinatal HIV-1 transmission in the United States. *Morbid Mortal Weekly Rep* 2002;51(RR-18):1–38
11. Durand ML, Calderwood SB, Weber DJ, *et al*. Acute bacterial meningitis in adults: a review of 493 episodes. *N Engl J Med* 1993;328:21–8
12. Quagliarello VJ, Scheld M. Treatment of bacterial meningitis. *N Engl J Med* 1997;336:708–16

13. Schuchat A, Robinson K, Wenger JD, *et al.* Bacterial meningitis in the United States in 1995. *N Engl J Med* 1997;337:970–6
14. Duff P. Antibiotic selection in obstetric patients. *Infect Dis Clin North Am* 1997;11:1–10
15. Duff P. Antibiotic selection in obstetrics: making cost-effective choices. *Clin Obstet Gynecol* 2002;45:59–72
16. Luby JP. Southwestern Internal Medicine conference: infections of the central nervous system. *Am J Med Sci* 1992;304:379–91
17. Estanislao LB, Pachner AR. Spirochetal infection of the nervous system. *Neurol Clin* 1999;17:783–800
18. Boucher M, Yonekura ML. Listeria meningitis during pregnancy. *Am J Perinatol* 1984;1:312–18
19. Figueroa R, Bracero LA, Aguero-Rosenfeld M, *et al.* Confirmation of *Borrelia burgdorferi spirochetes* by polymerase chain reaction in placentas of women with reactive serology for Lyme antibodies. *Gynecol Obstet Invest* 1996;41:240–3
20. Mikkelsen AL, Palle C. Lyme disease during pregnancy. *Acta Obstet Gynecol Scand* 1987;66:477–8
21. Elliott DJ, Eppes SC, Klein JD. Teratogen update: Lyme disease. *Teratology* 2001;64:276–81
22. Shapiro ED, Gerber MA. Lyme disease: fact versus fiction. *Pediatr Ann* 2002;31:170–7
23. Strobino BA, Williams CL, Abid S, *et al.* Lyme disease and pregnancy outcome: a prospective study of two thousand prenatal patients. *Am J Obstet Gynecol* 1993;169:367 71
24. Strobino B, Abid S, Gewitz M. Maternal Lyme disease and congenital heart disease: a case–control study in an endemic area. *Am J Obstet Gynecol* 1999;180:711–16
25. Centers for Disease Control. Primary and secondary syphilis – United States, 2000–2001. *Morbid Mortal Weekly Rep* 2002;51:971–4
26. Chen CP, Wang KG. Cryptococcal meningitis in pregnancy. *Am J Perinatol* 1996;13:35–6
27. Clark WC, Metcalf JC, Muhlbauer MS, *et al. Mycobacterium tuberculosis* meningitis: a report of twelve cases and a literature review. *Neurosurgery* 1986:18:604–10
28. Ely EW, Peacock JE, Haponik EF, *et al.* Cryptococcal pneumonia complicating pregnancy. *Medicine* 1998;77:153–67
29. Hamadeh MA, Glassroth J. Tuberculosis and pregnancy. *Chest* 1992;101: 1114–20
30. Petrini B, Gentz J, Winbladh B, *et al.* Perinatal transmission of tuberculosis: meningitis in mother, disseminated disease in child. *Scand J Infect Dis* 1983;15:403–5
31. Pereira CA, Fischman O, Colombo Al, *et al.* Cryptococcal meningitis in pregnancy. Review of the literature. Report of 2 cases. *Rev Inst Med Trop Sao Paulo* 1993;35:367–71
32. Peterson CM, Schuppert K, Kelly PC, *et al.* Coccidioidomycosis and pregnancy. *Obstet Gynecol Surv* 1993;48:149–56

33. Lee BE, Feinberg M, Abraham JJ, *et al.* Congenital malformations in an infant born to a woman treated with fluconazole. *Pediatr Infect Dis* 1992; 11:1062–4
34. Hankey GJ, Bucens MR, Chambers JSW. Herpes simplex encephalitis in third trimester of pregnancy: successful outcome for mother and child. *Neurology* 1987;37:1534–7
35. Centers for Disease Control. Provisional surveillance summary of the West Nile virus epidemic – United States, January–November 2002. *Morbid Mortal Weekly Rep* 2002;51:1129–33
36. Centers for Disease Control. Intrauterine West Nile virus infection – New York, 2002. *Morbid Mortal Weekly Rep* 2002;51:1135–6
37. Stagno S, Whitley RJ. Herpes virus infection of pregnancy. Part I. Cytomegalovirus and Epstein–Barr virus infection. *N Engl J Med* 1984; 313:1270–4
38. Mendizabal JE, Bassam BA. Guillain–Barré syndrome and cytomegalovirus infection during pregnancy. *South Med Assoc J* 1997;90:63–4
39. Costa S, Barrasso R, Terzano P, *et al.* Detection of active Epstein–Barr infection in pregnant women. *Eur J Clin Microbiol* 1985;4:335–6
40. Causer LM, Newman RD, Barber AM, *et al.* Malaria surveillance – United States, 2000. *Morbid Mortal Weekly Rep* 2002;51(SS-5):9–21
41. Alger LS. Toxoplasmosis and parvovirus B12. *Infect Dis Clin North Am* 1997;11:55–75
42. Willis MS, Southern P, Latimer MJ. *Toxoplasma* infection: making the best use of laboratory tests. *Infect Med* 2002;19:522–32
43. Forsgren M, Gille E, Jungstrom I, Nokes DJ. *Toxoplasma gondii* antibodies in pregnant women in Stockholm in 1969, 1979 and 1987. *Lancet* 1991; 337:1413–14
44. Wong S-Y, Remington JS. Toxoplasmosis in pregnancy. *Clin Infect Dis* 1993;18:853–62
45. Hohlfeld P, Daffos F, Costa J-M, *et al.* Prenatal diagnosis of congenital toxoplasmosis with a polymerase-chain-reaction test on amniotic fluid. *N Engl J Med* 1994;331:685–99
46. Holliman RE. Congenital toxoplasmosis: prevention, screening and treatment. *J Hosp Infect* 1995;30(Suppl):179–90
47. Kurl R, Montella KR. Cysticercosis as a cause of seizure disorder in pregnancy: case report and review of literature. *Am J Perinatol* 1994;11: 409–11
48. Wheeler D, Keiser P, Rigamonti D, *et al.* Medical management of spinal epidural abscesses: case report and review. *Clin Infect Dis* 1992;15:22–7
49. Cheng Q, Jiang GX, Fredrickson S, *et al.* Increased incidence of Guillain–Barré syndrome postpartum. *Epidemiology* 1998;9:601–4
50. Rolfs A, Bolik A. Guillain–Barré syndrome in pregnancy: reflections on immunopathogenesis. *Acta Neurol Scand* 1994;89:400–2
51. Smith JL. *Campylobacter jejuni* infection during pregnancy: long term consequences of associated bacteremia, Guillain–Barré syndrome and reactive arthritis. *J Food Protect* 2002;65:696–8
52. Fleisher G, Bolognese R. Epstein–Barr virus infection in pregnancy: a prospective study. *J Pediatr* 1984;104:374–9

Index